THE

40 MOST BEAUTIFUL
FLOWERS
IN THE WORLD

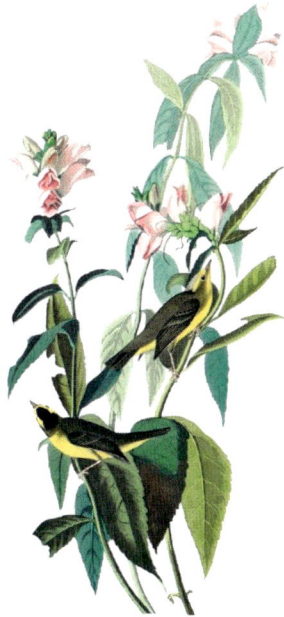

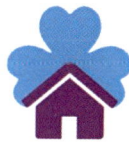

**BLUE CLOVER
BOOKS**

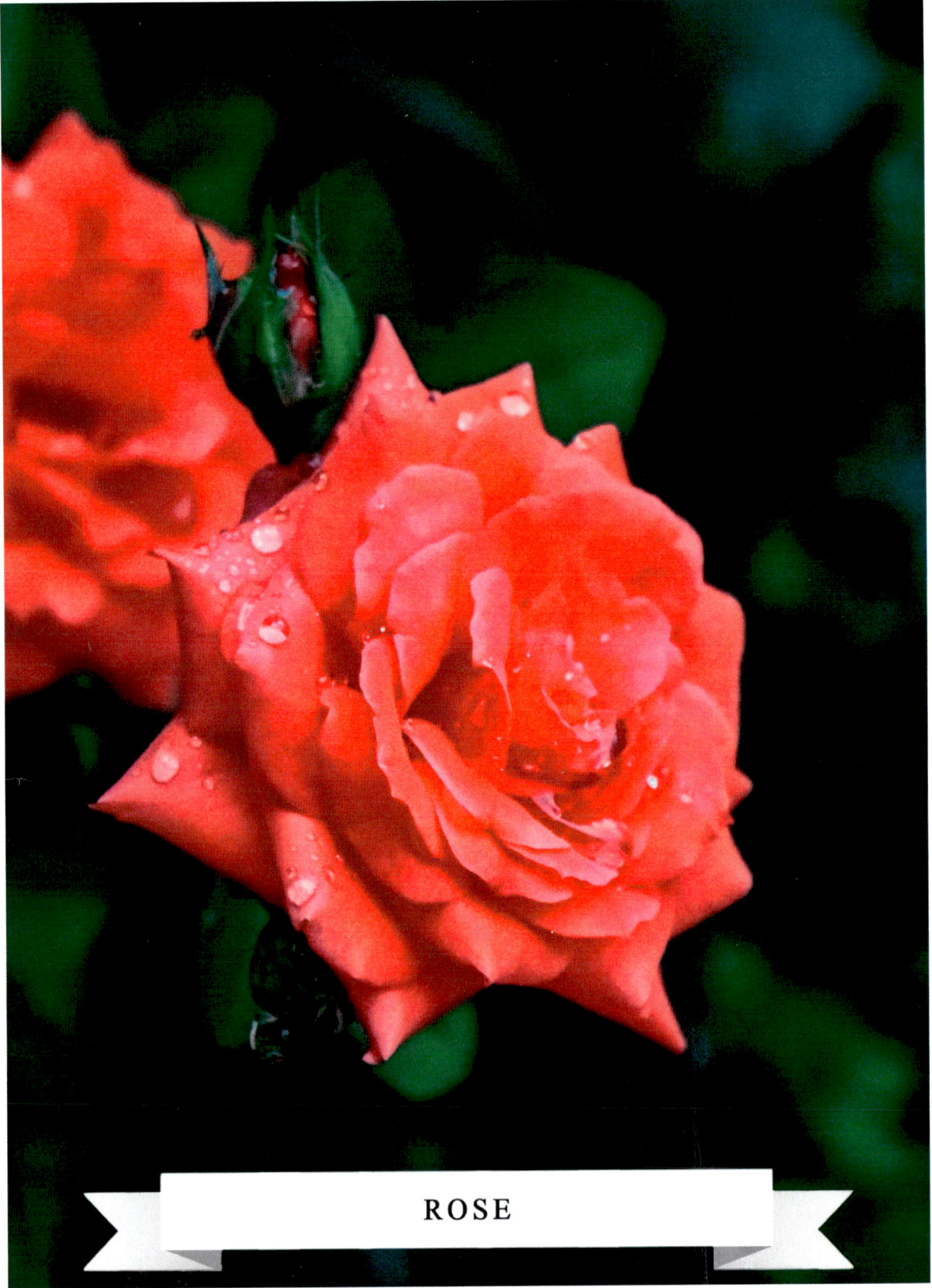

ROSE

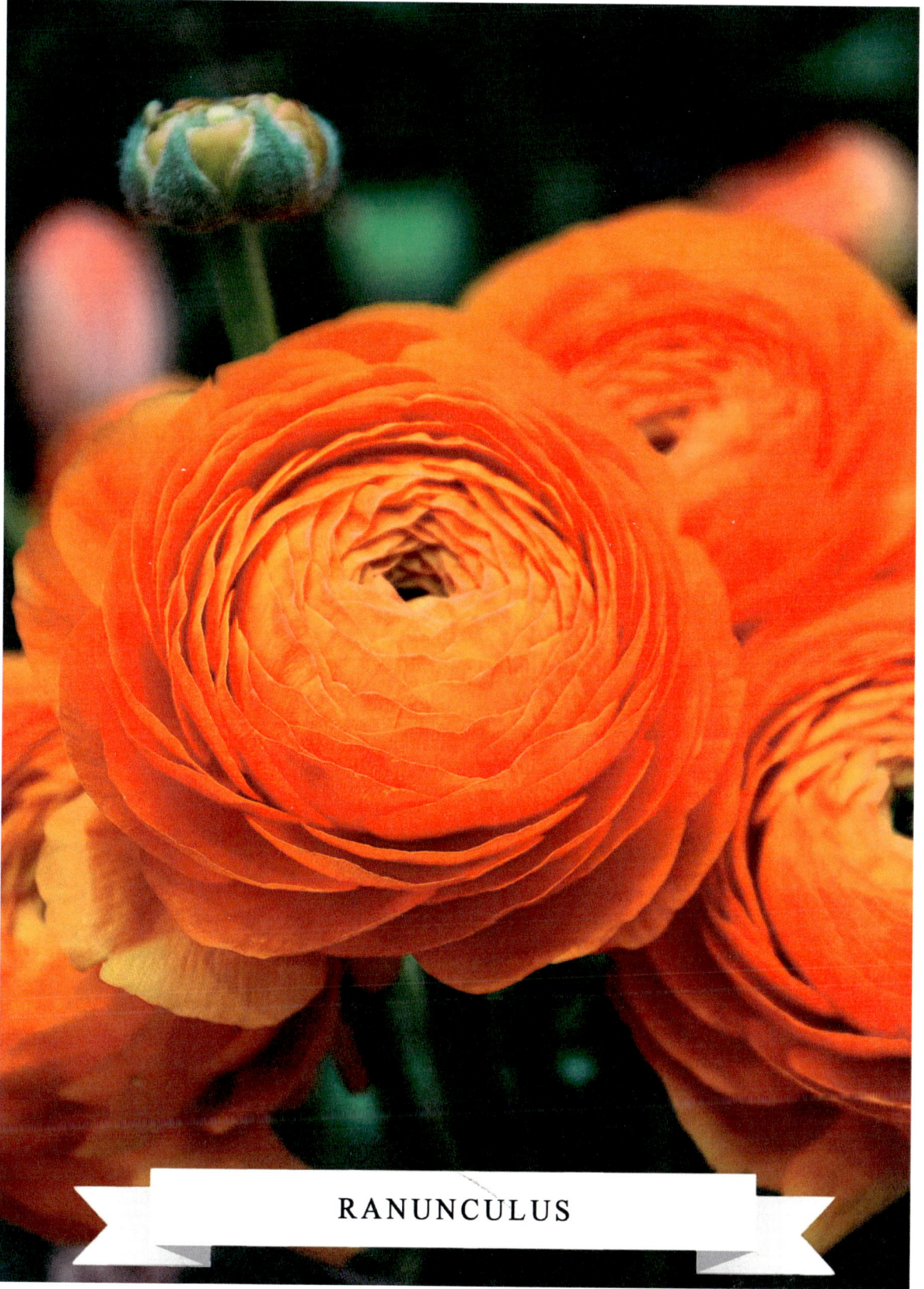

RANUNCULUS

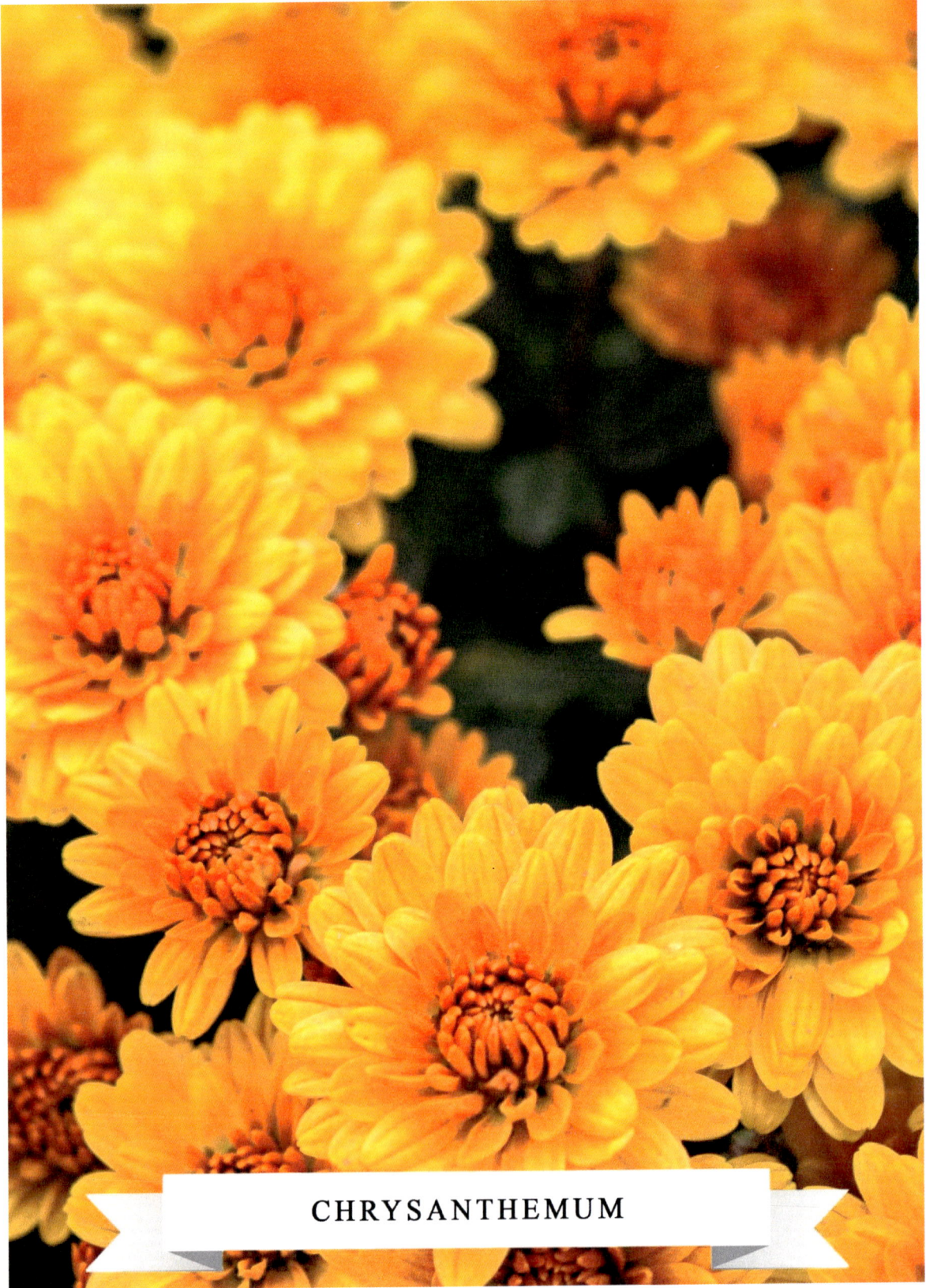

CHRYSANTHEMUM

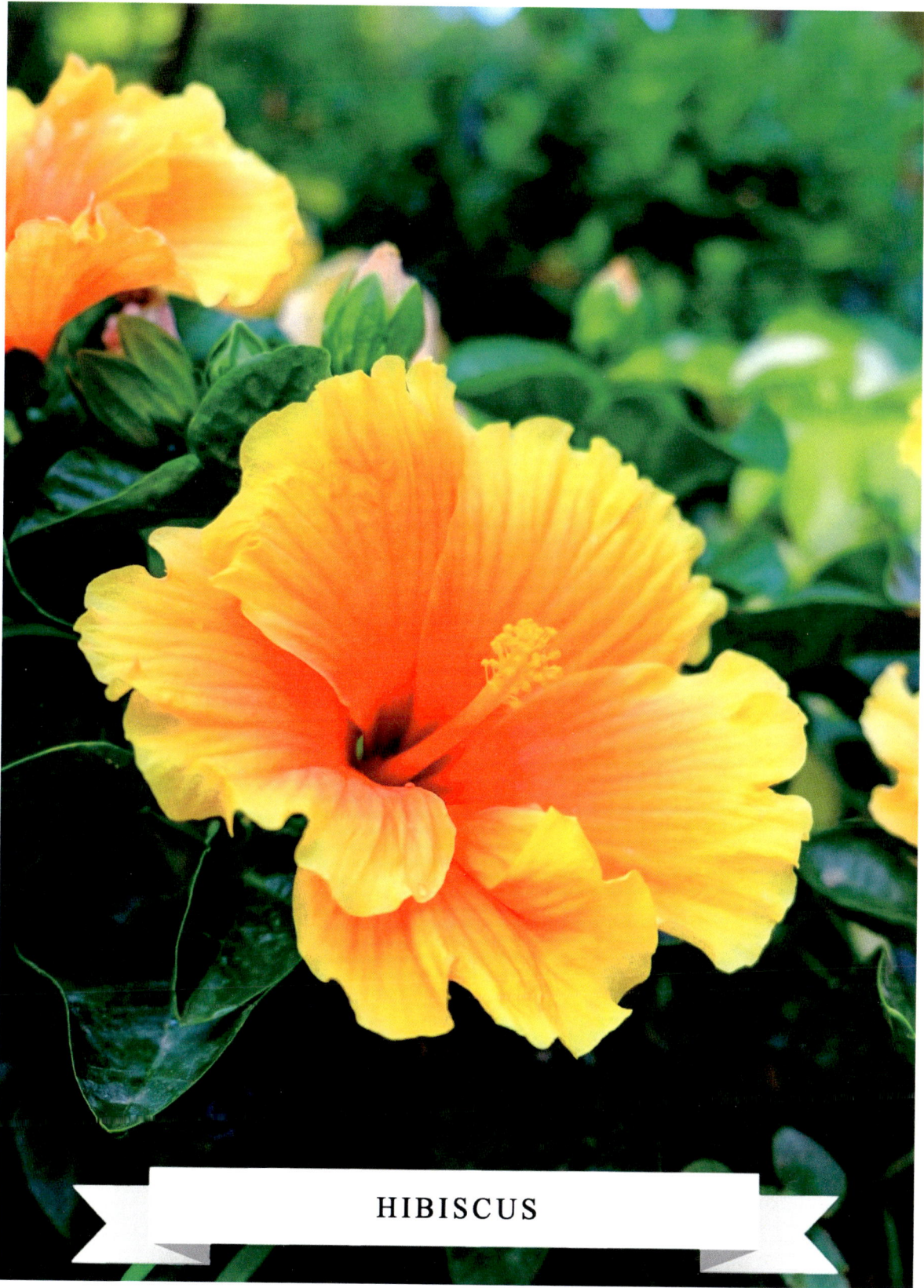

HIBISCUS

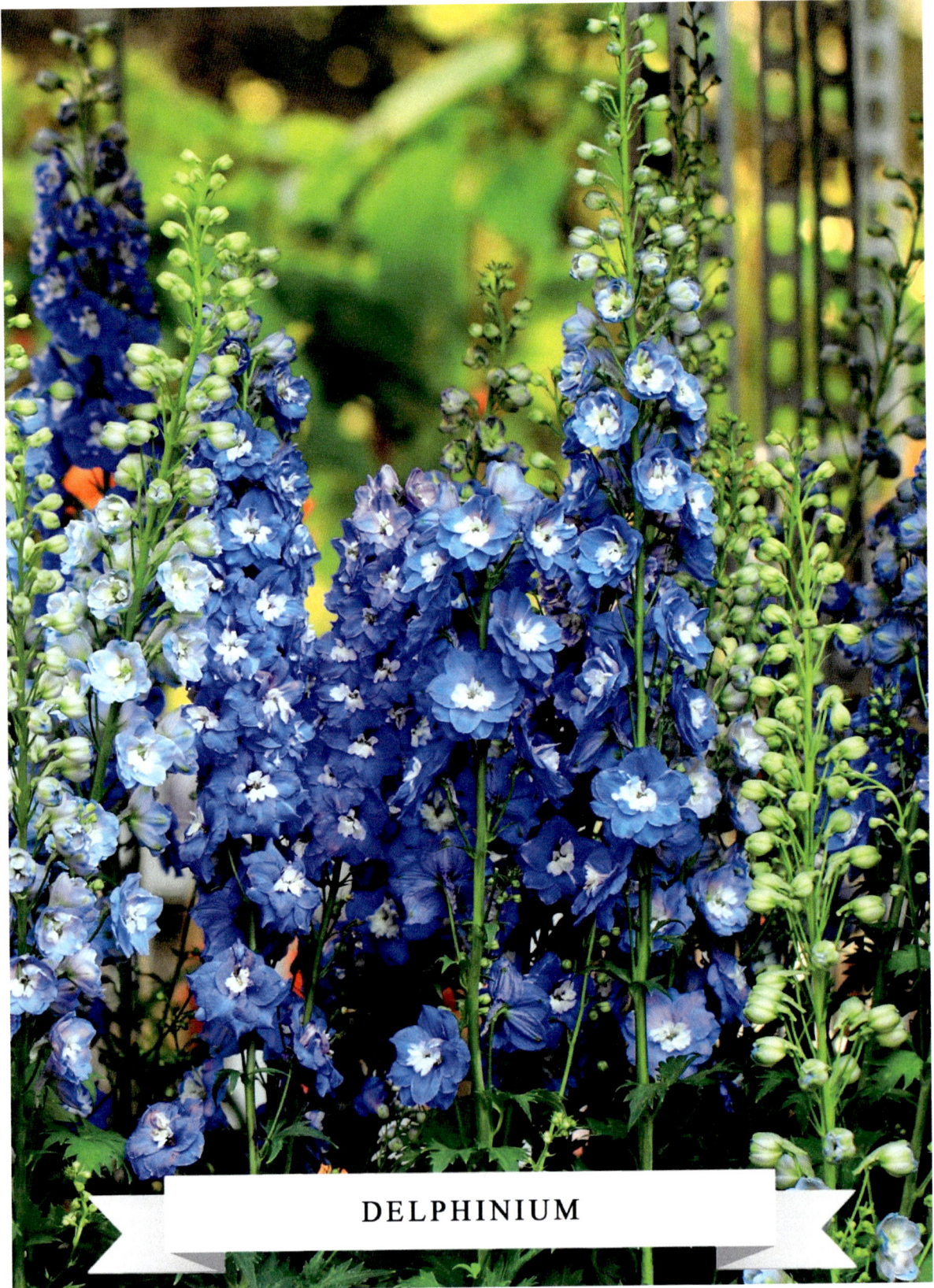

DELPHINIUM

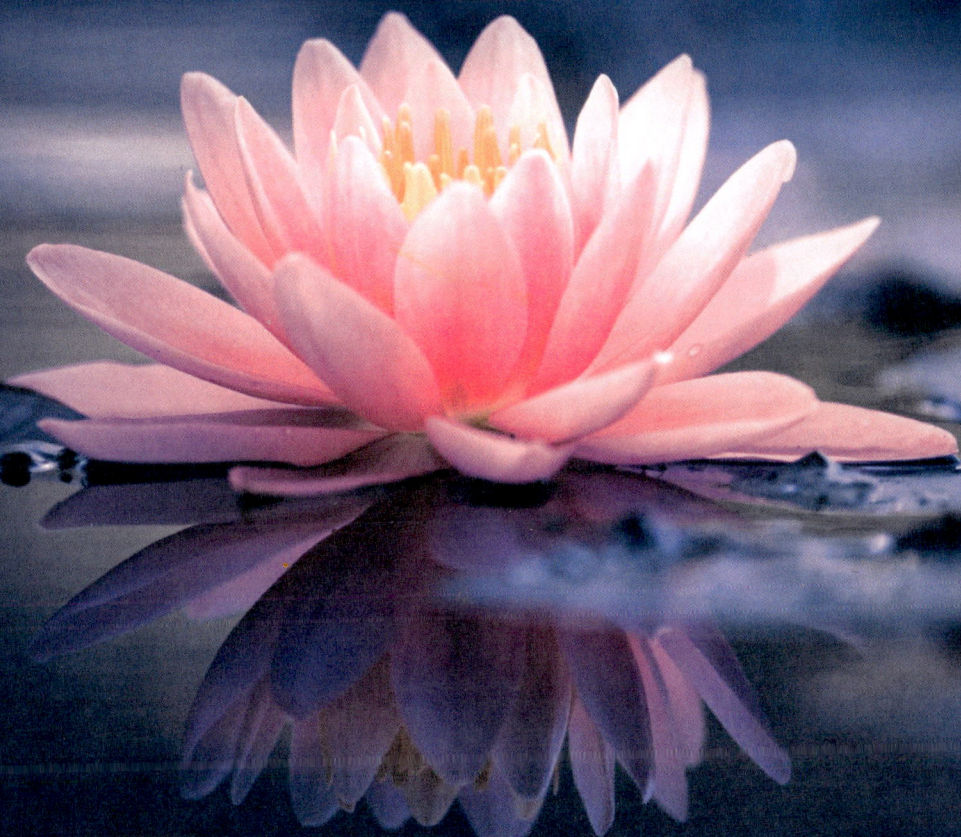

LOTUS

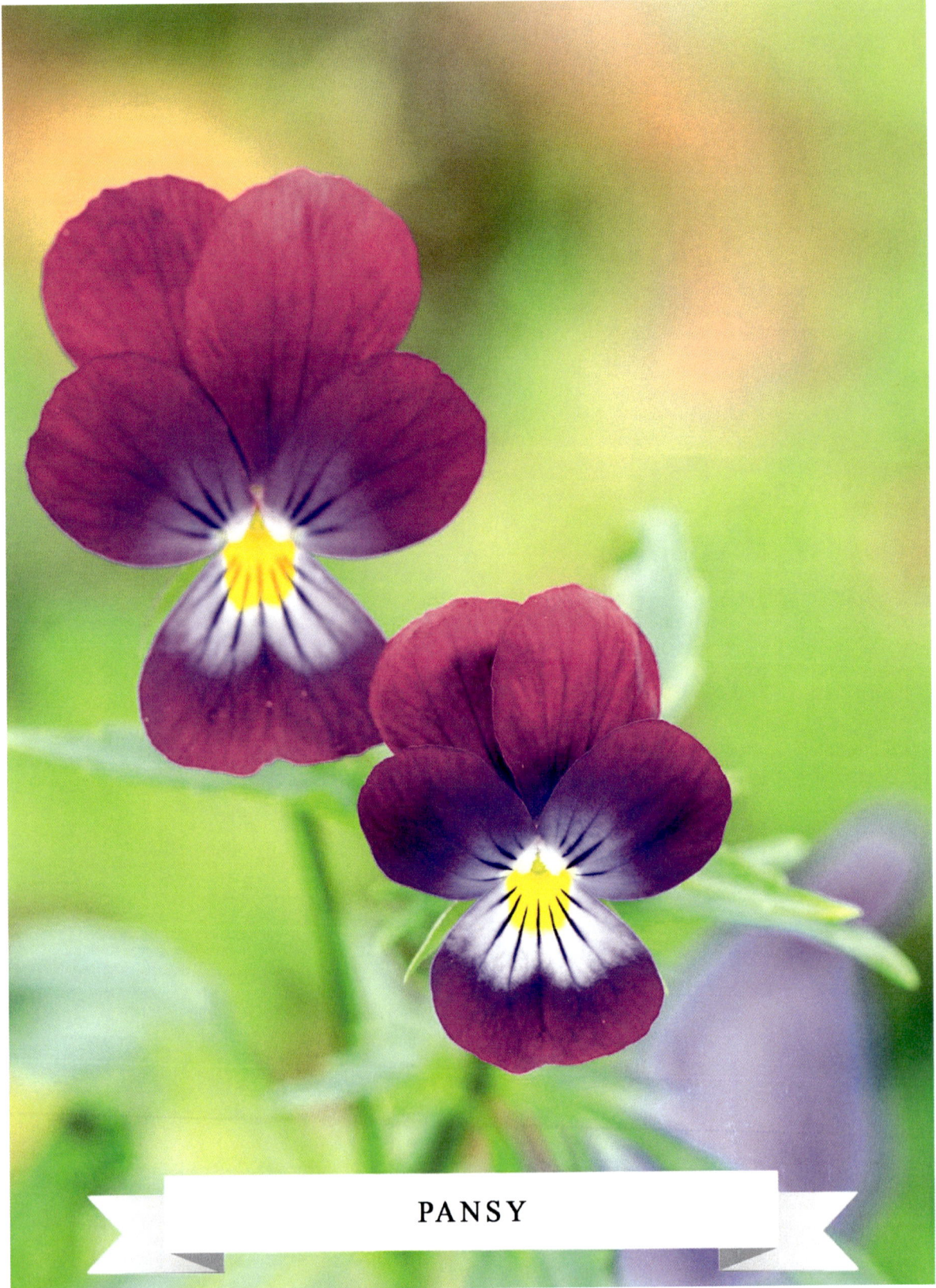

PANSY

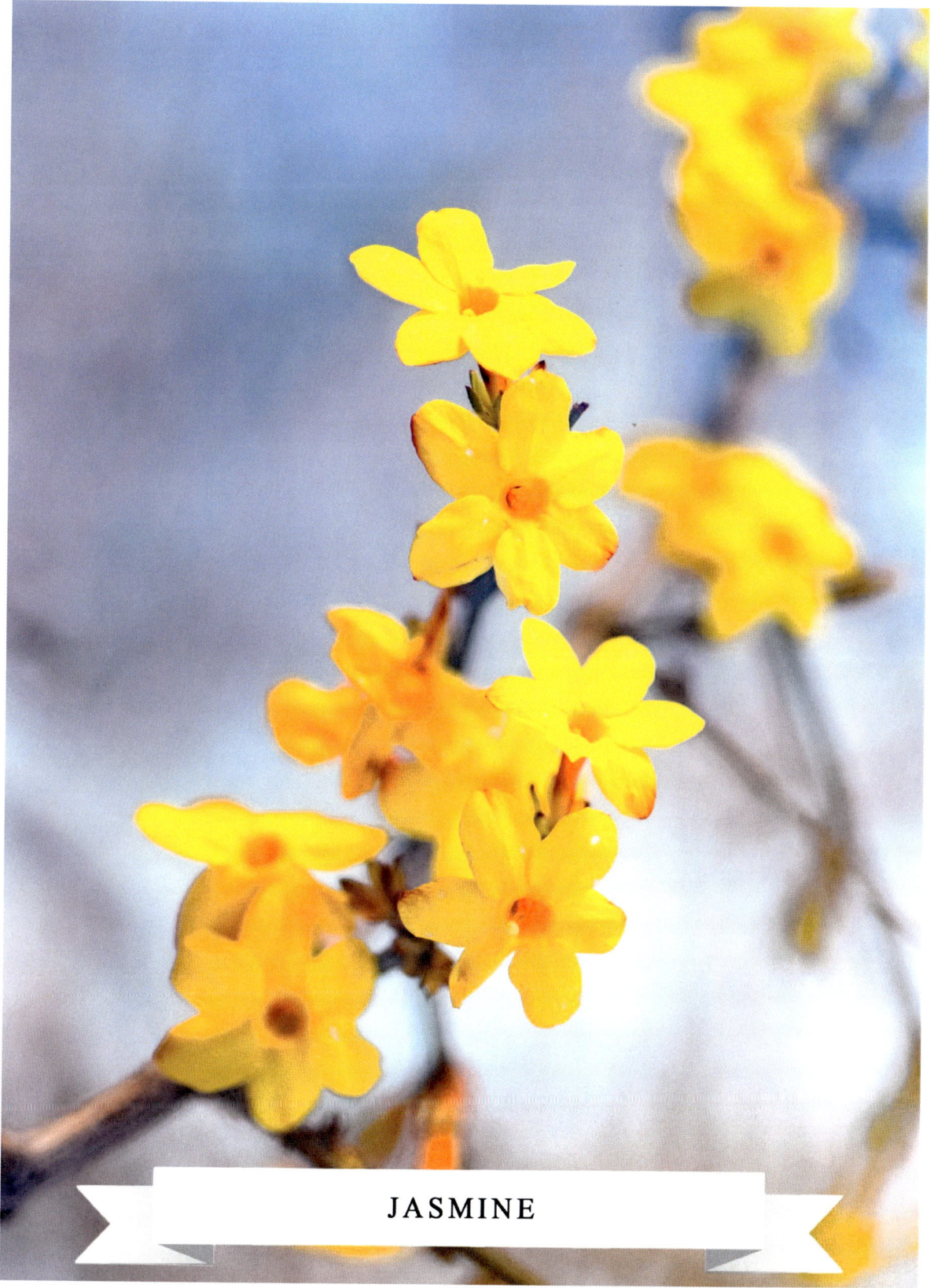

JASMINE

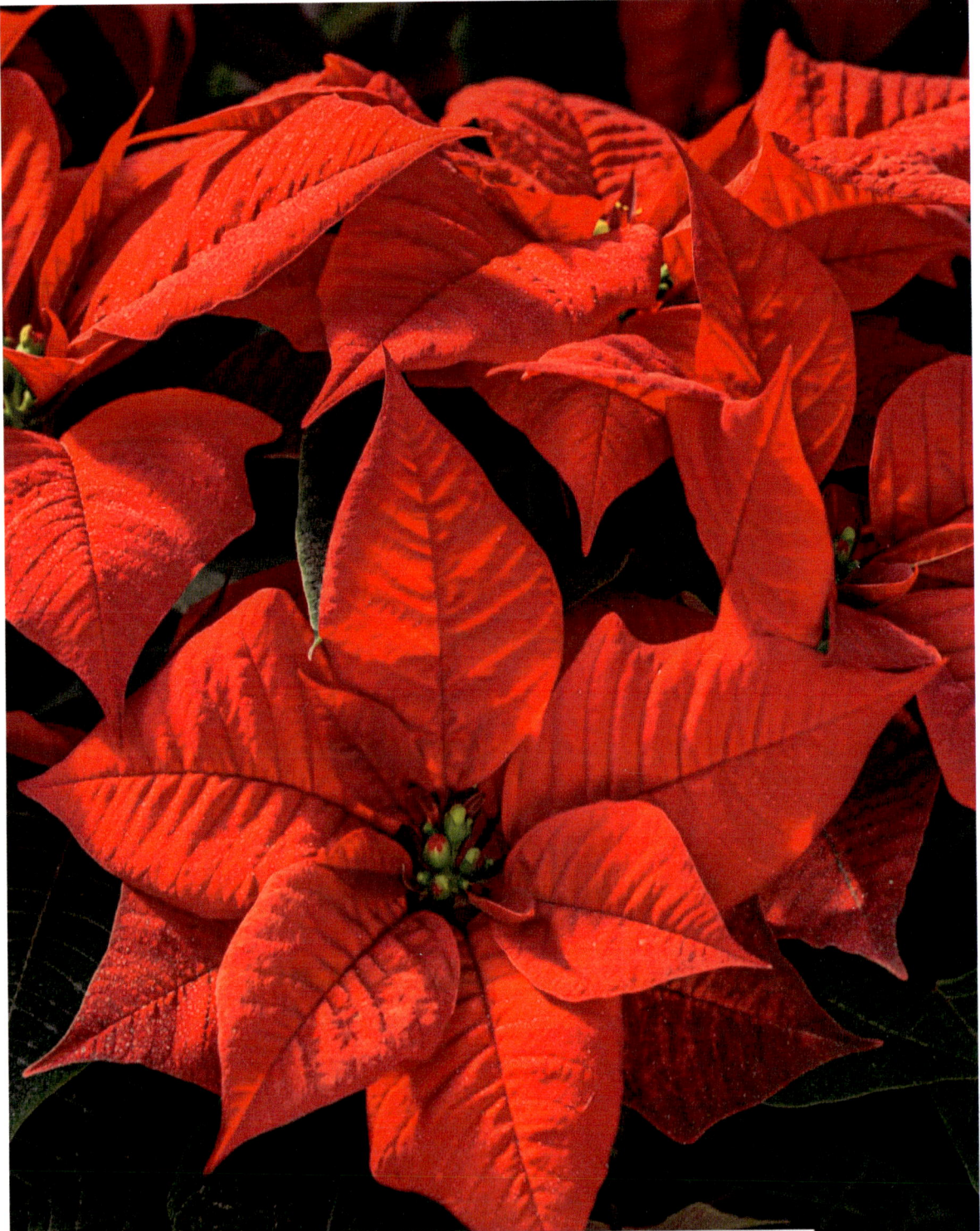

POINSETTIA

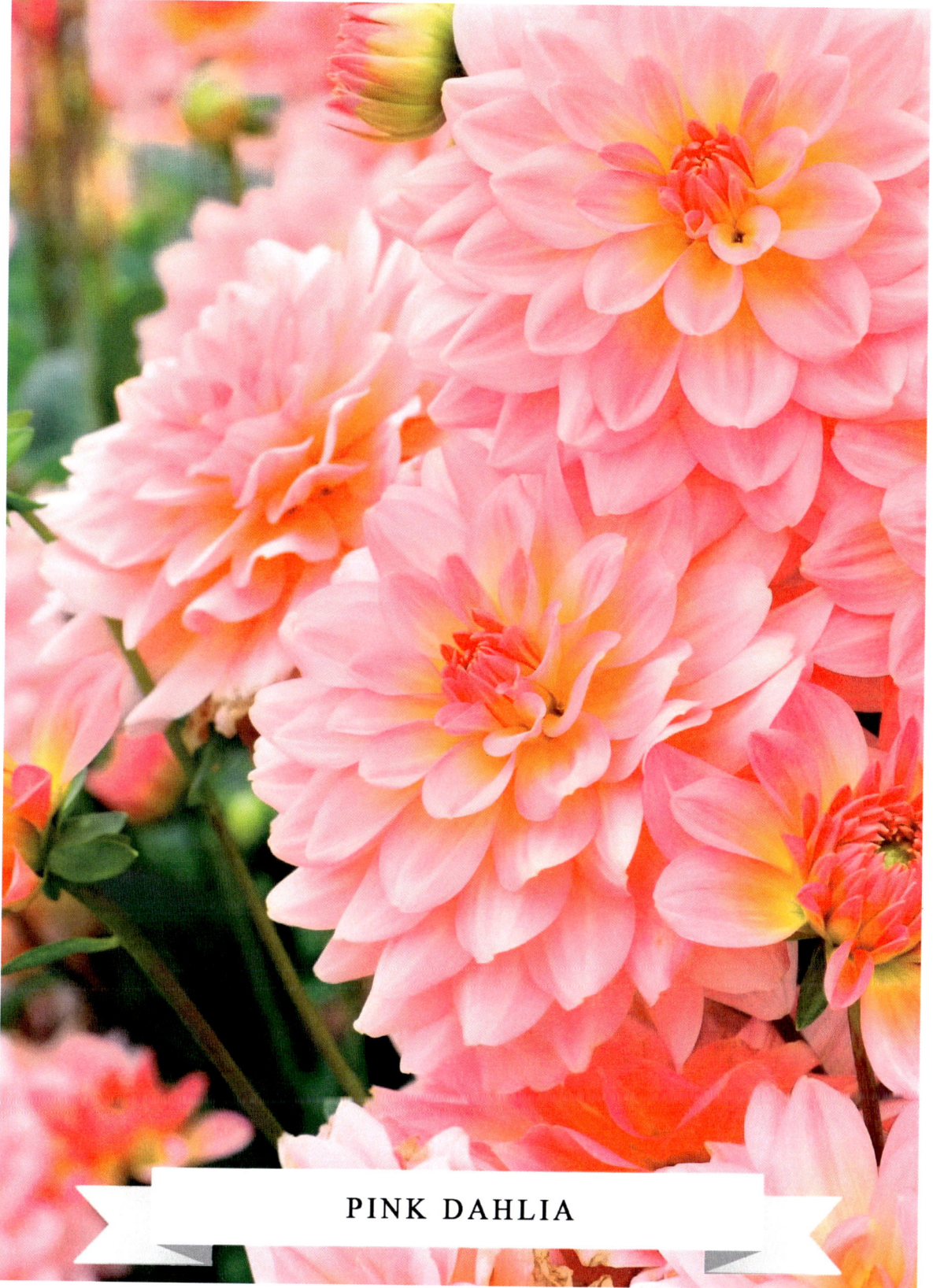

PINK DAHLIA

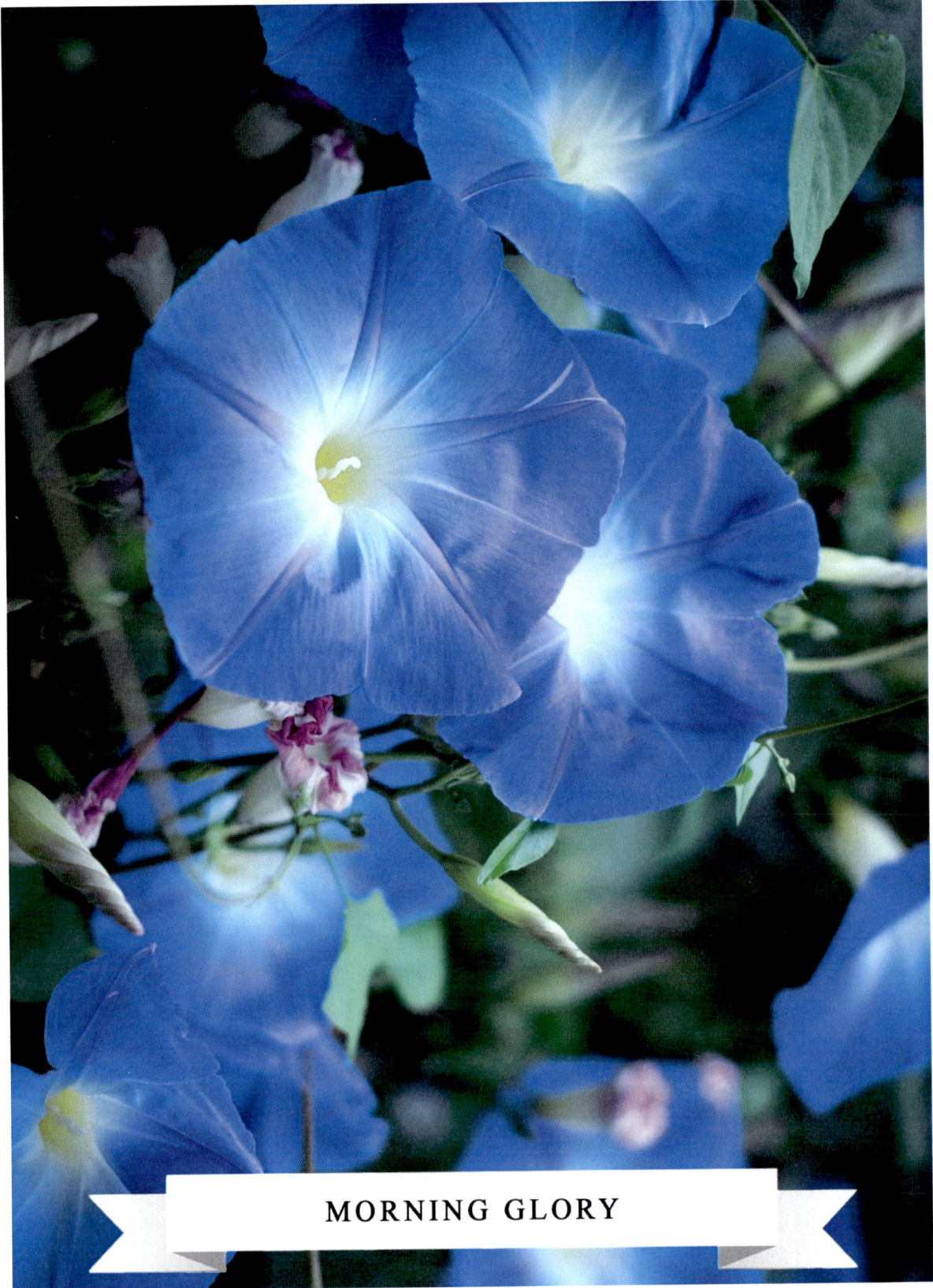

MORNING GLORY

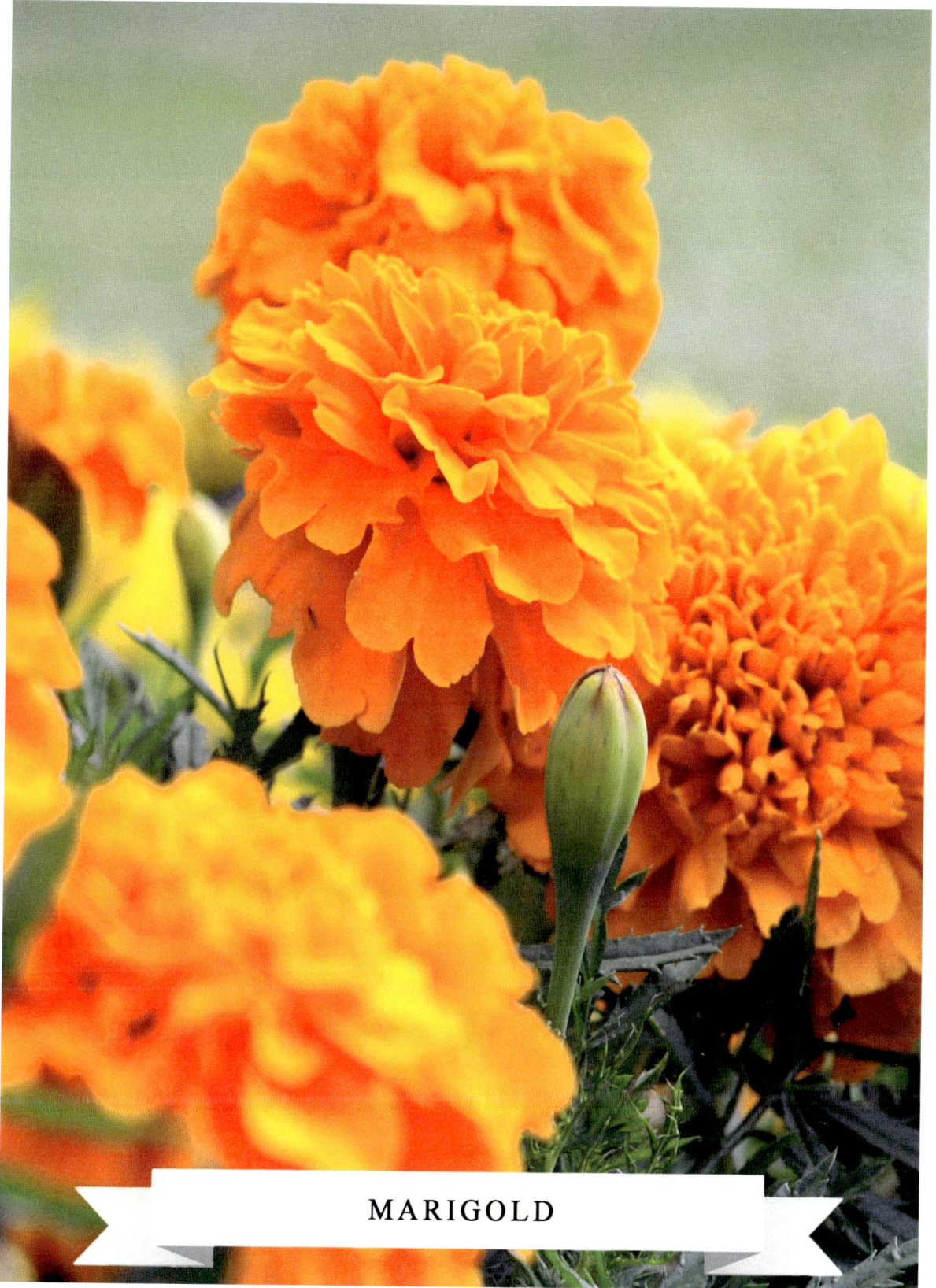

MARIGOLD

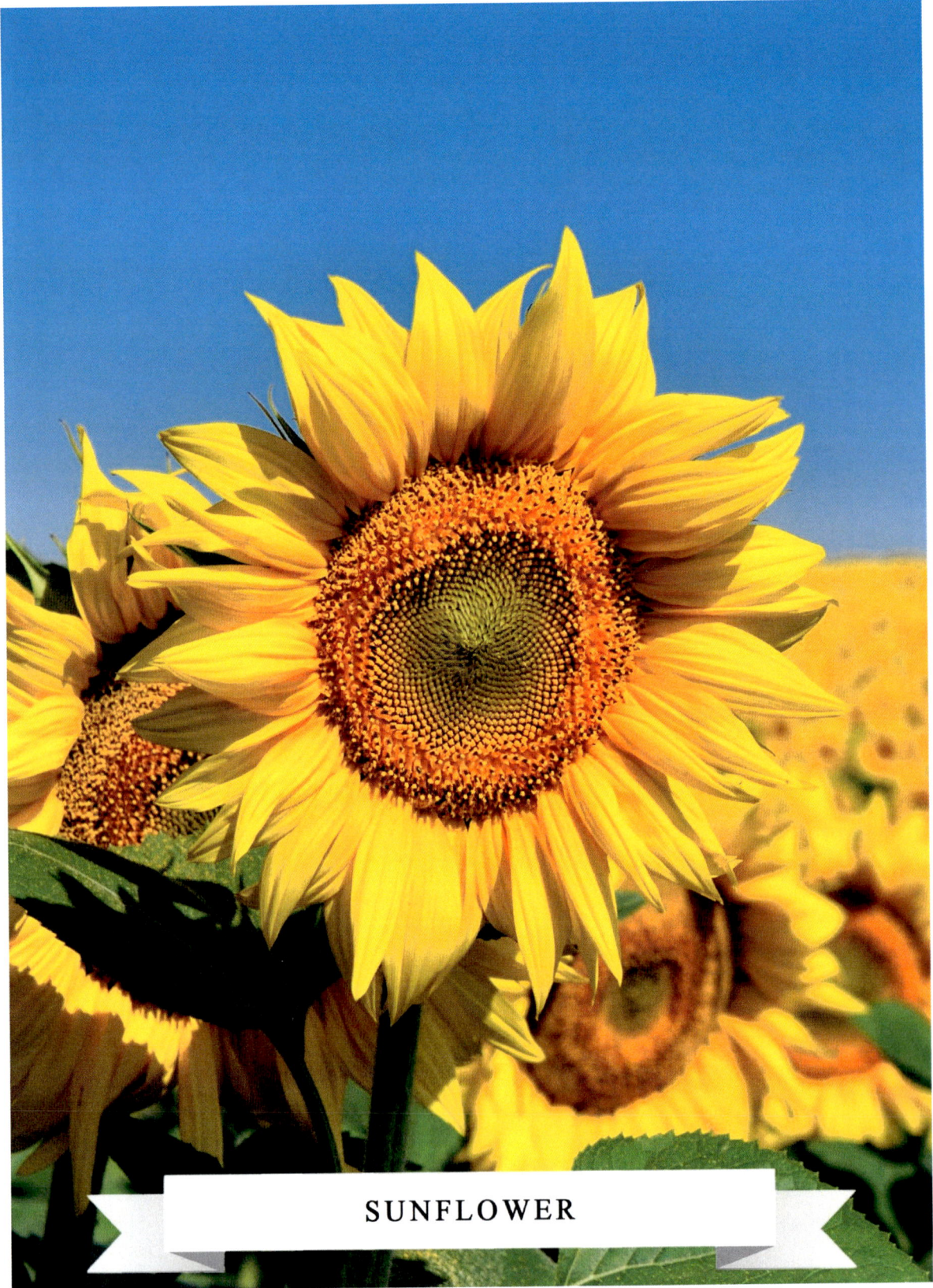

SUNFLOWER

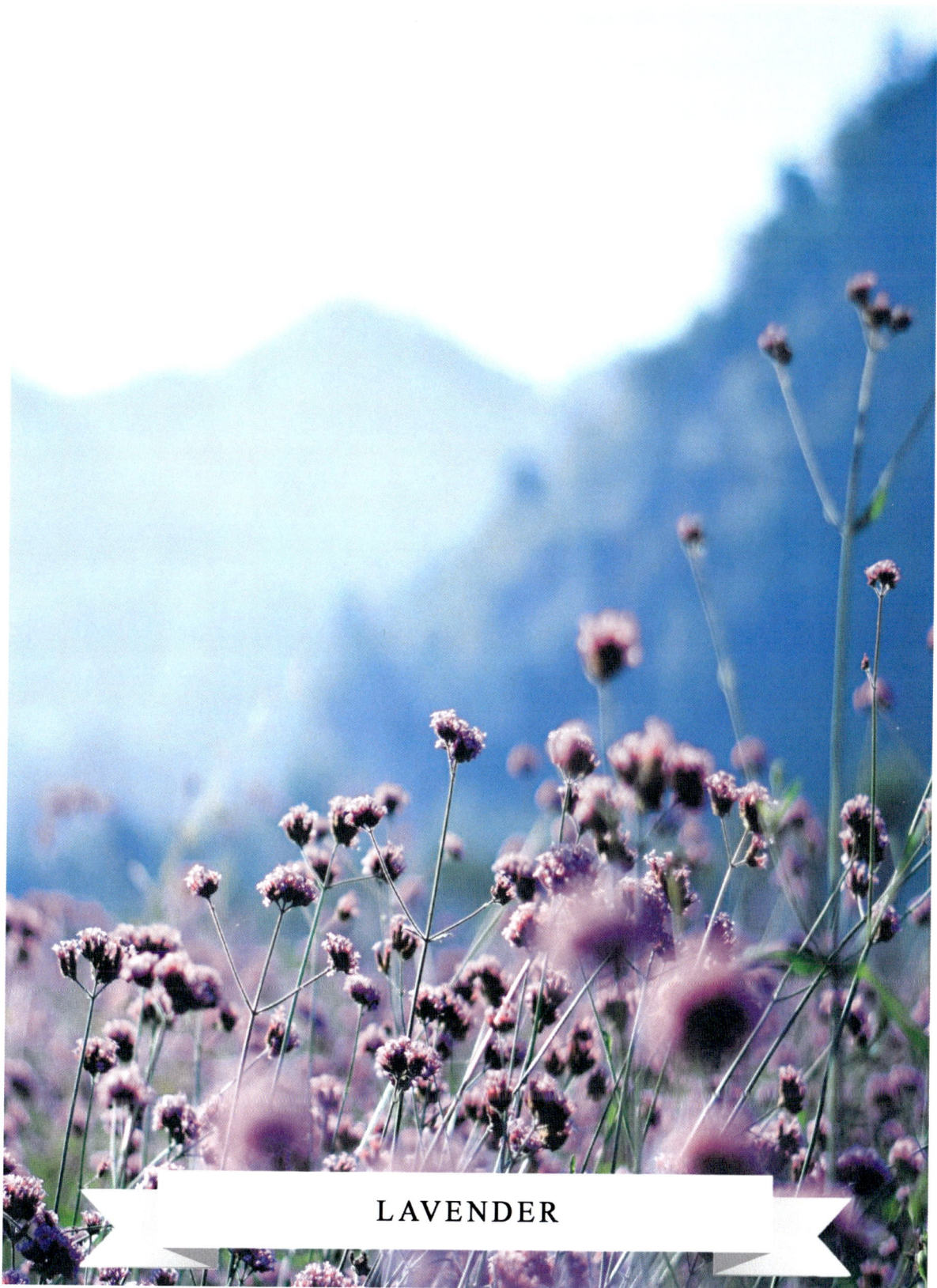

LAVENDER

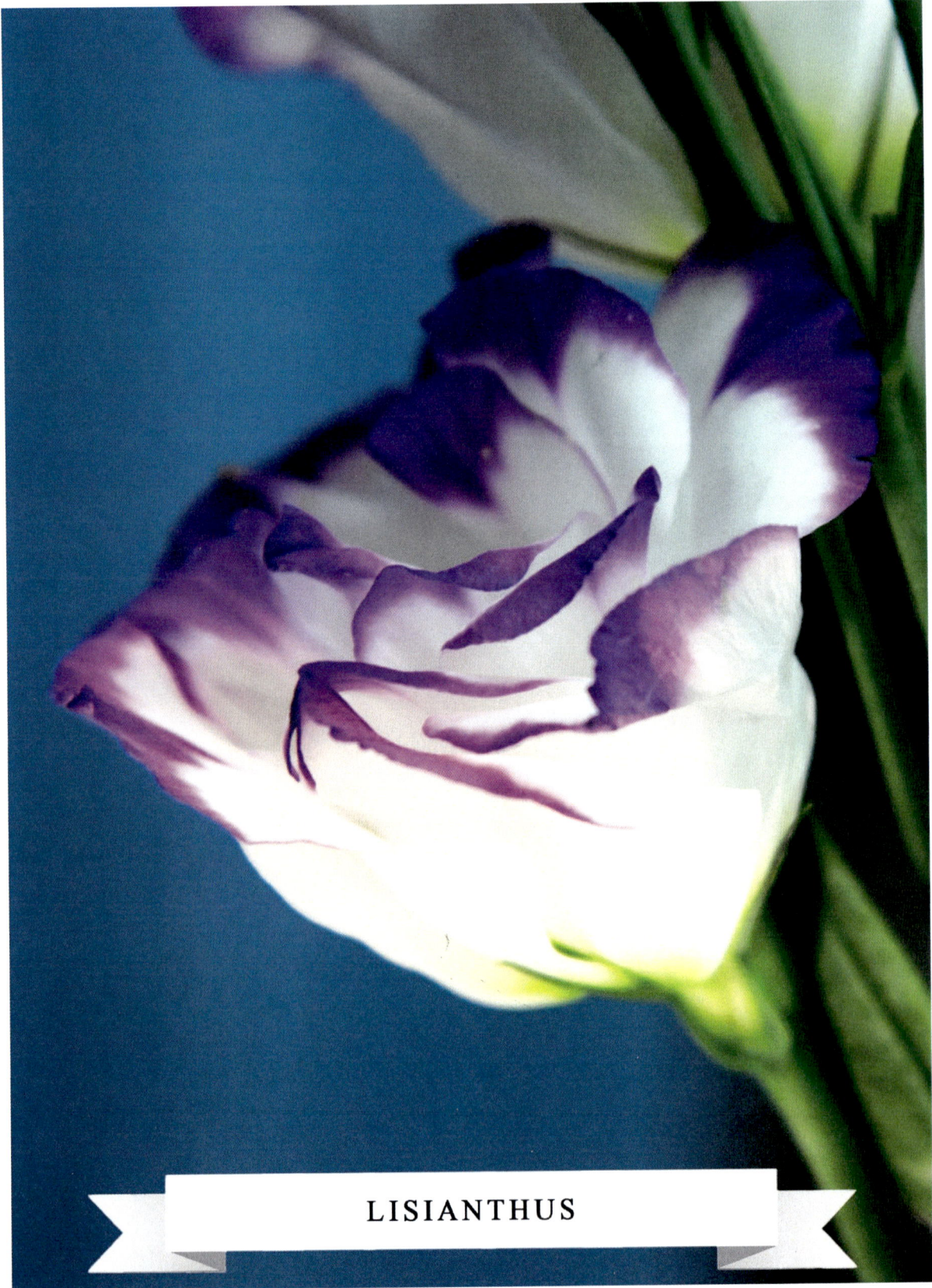

LISIANTHUS

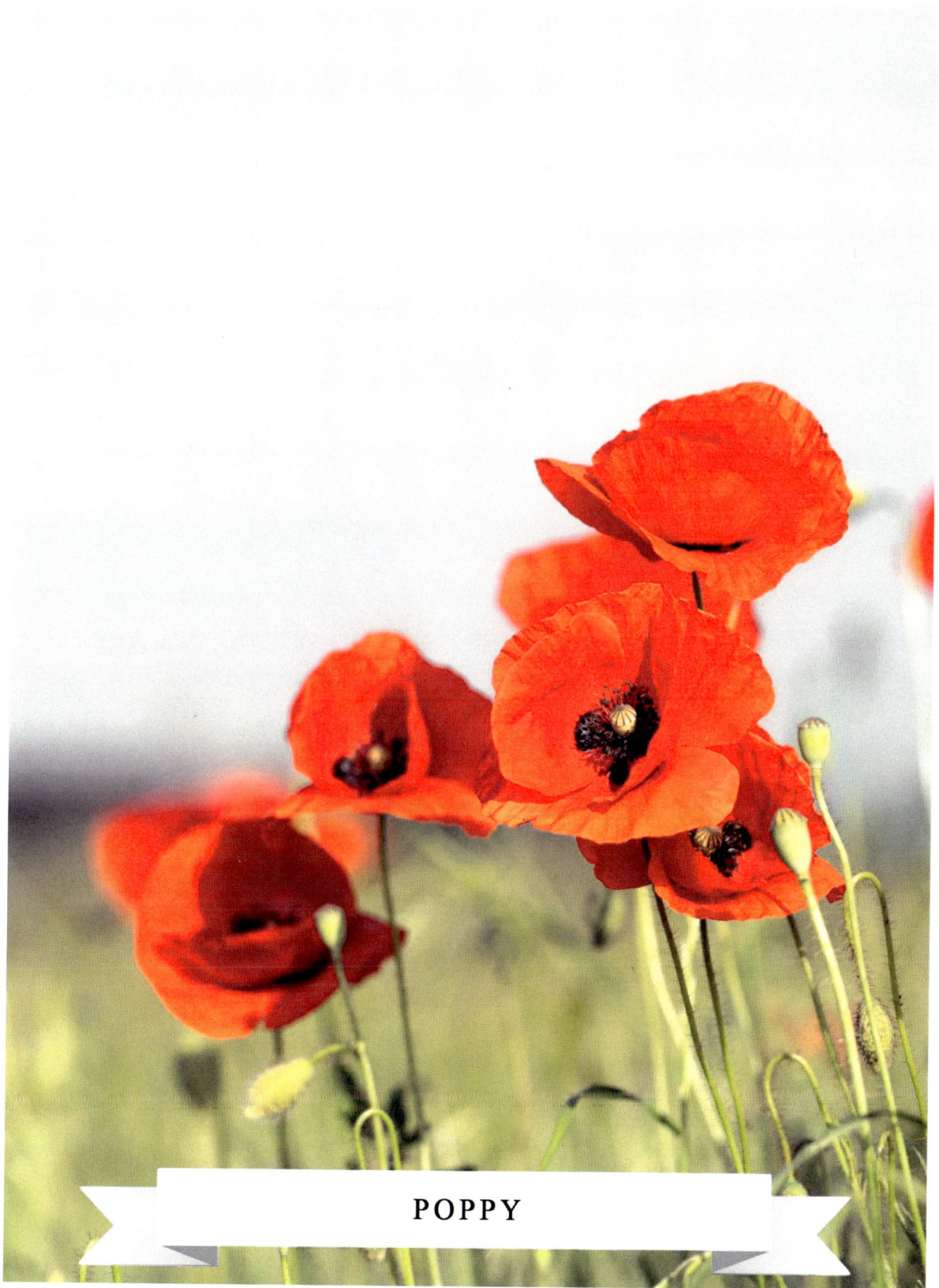

POPPY

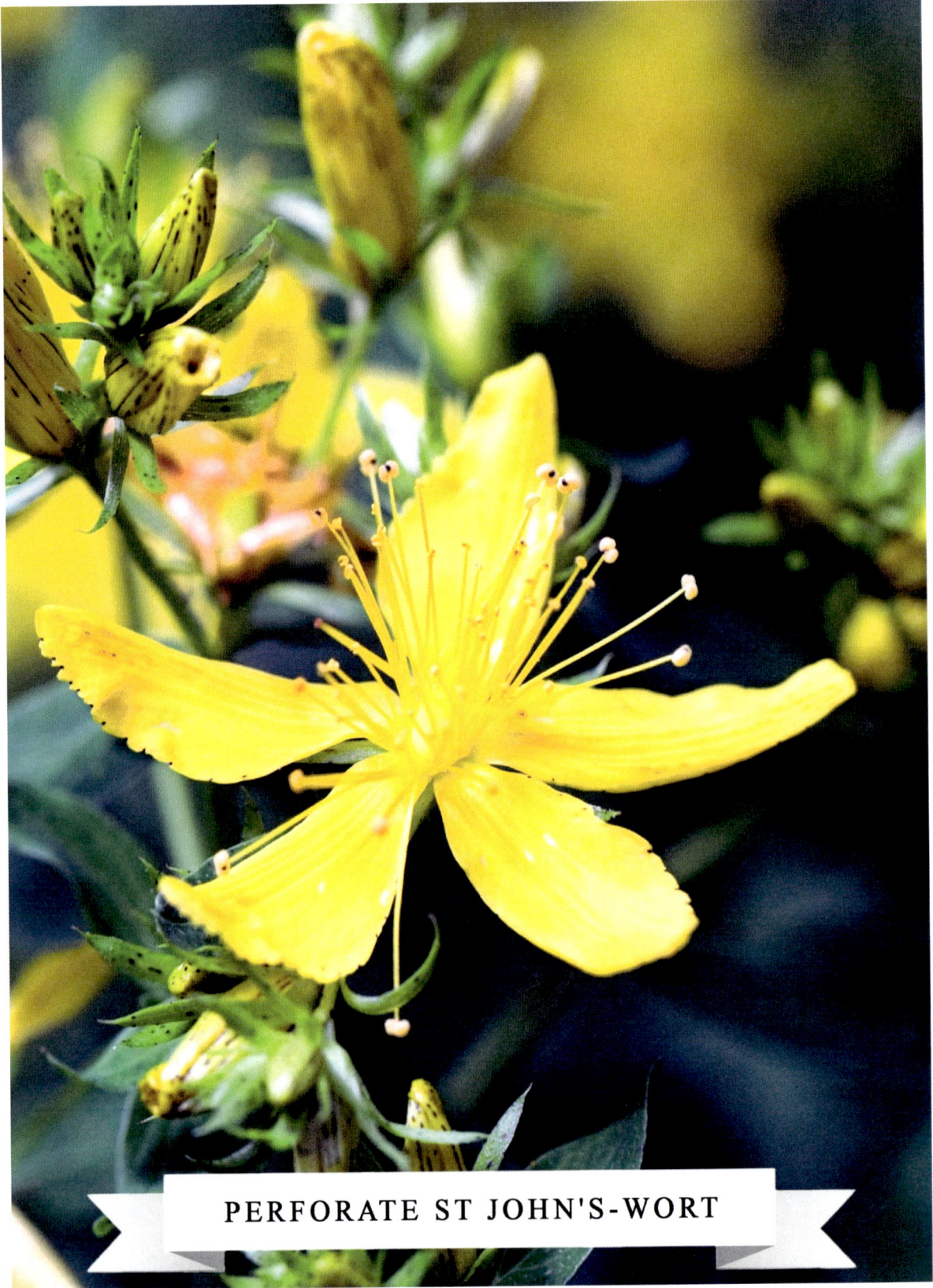

PERFORATE ST JOHN'S-WORT

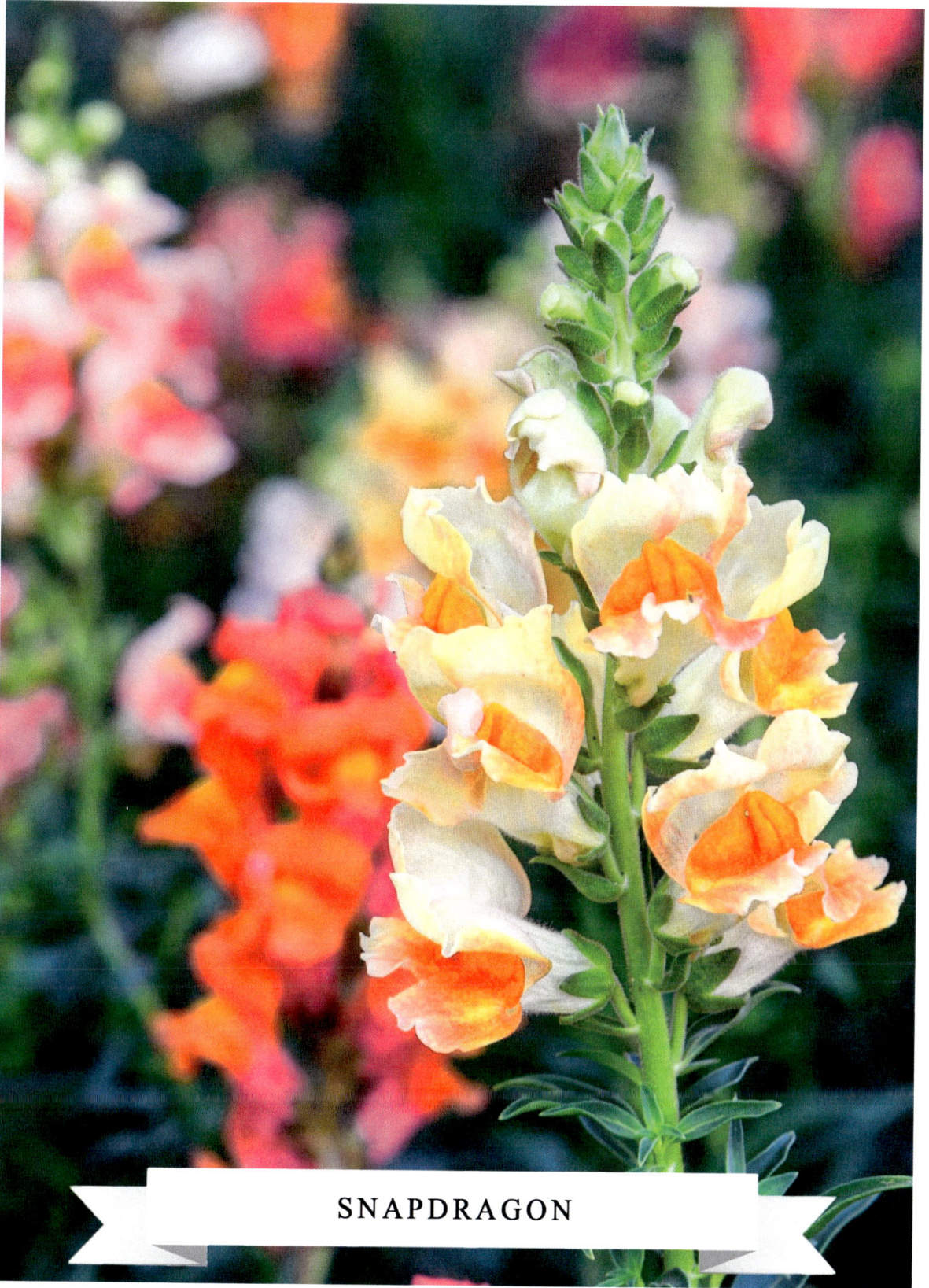

SNAPDRAGON

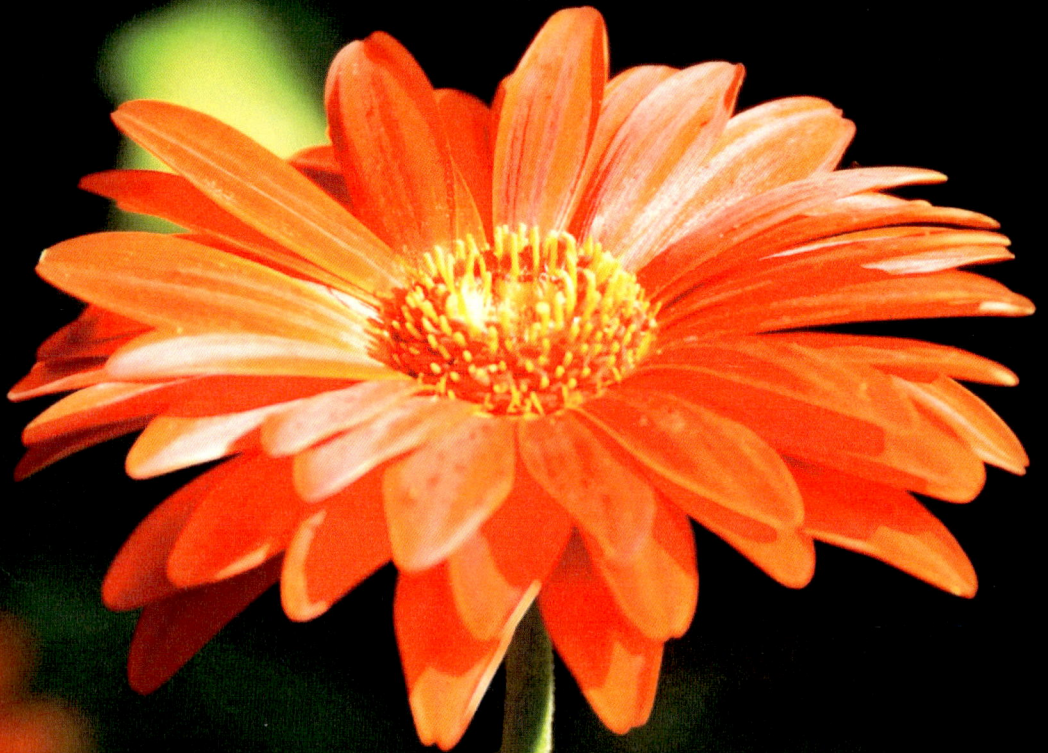

GERBERAS

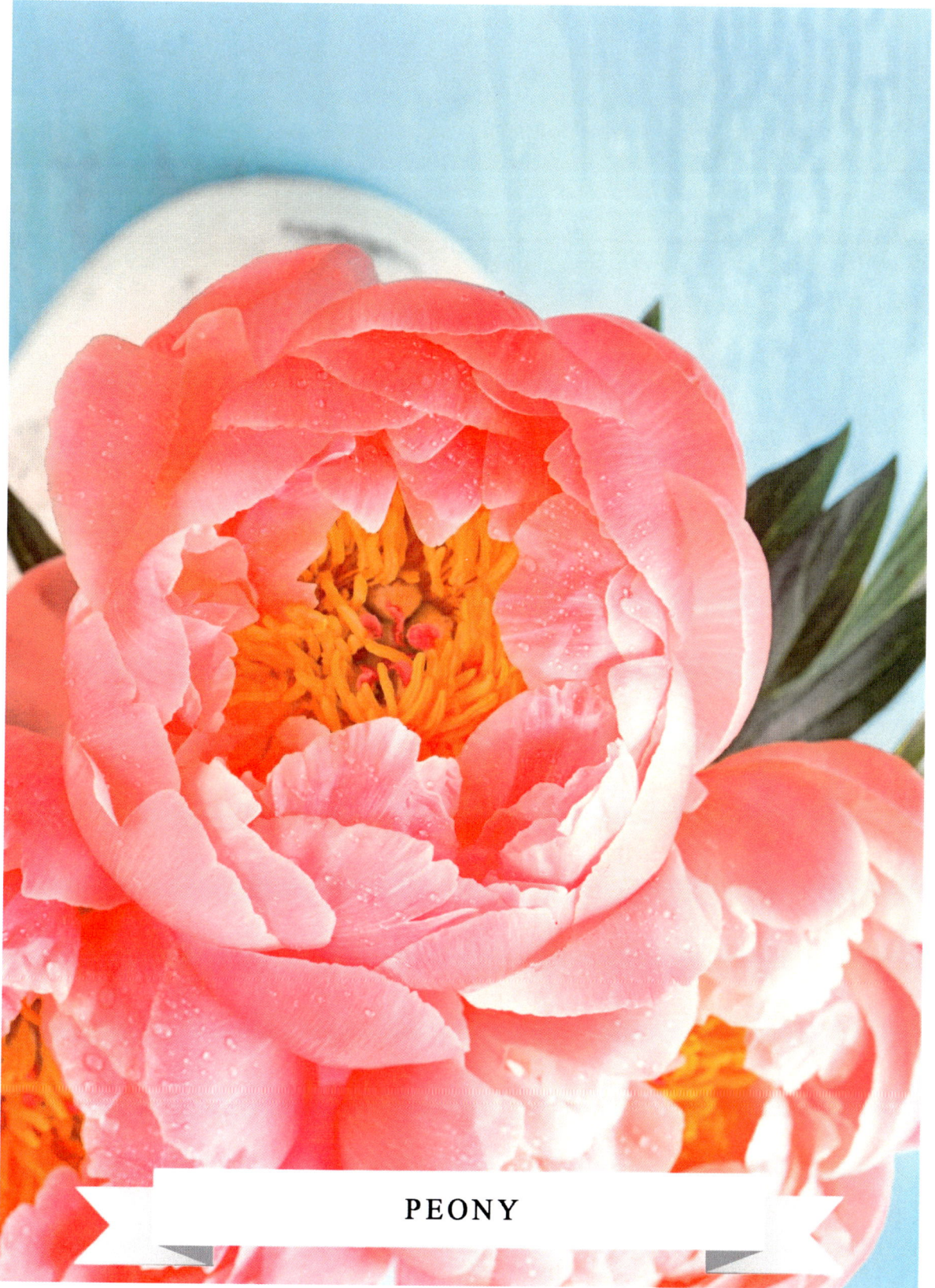

PEONY

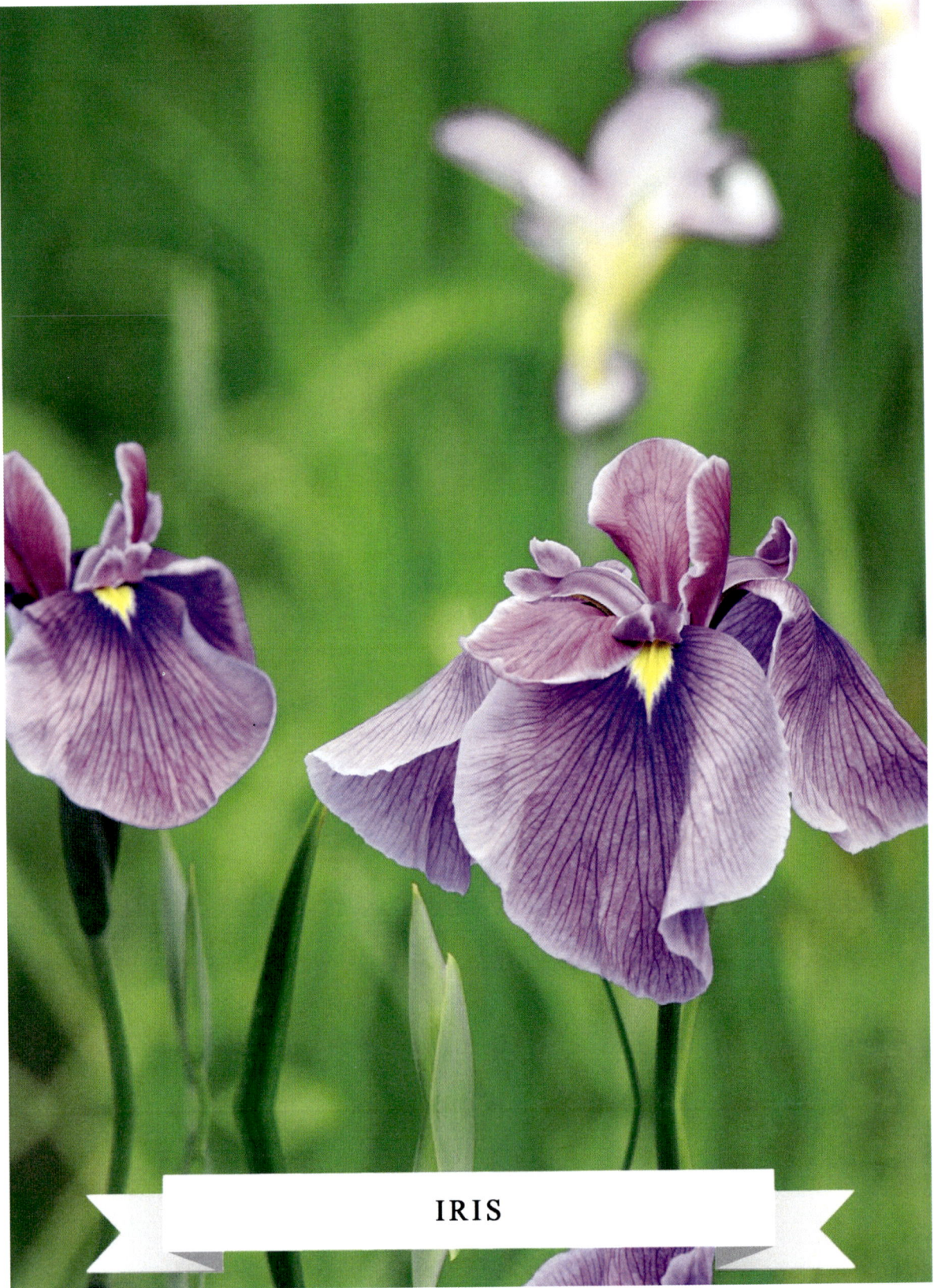

IRIS

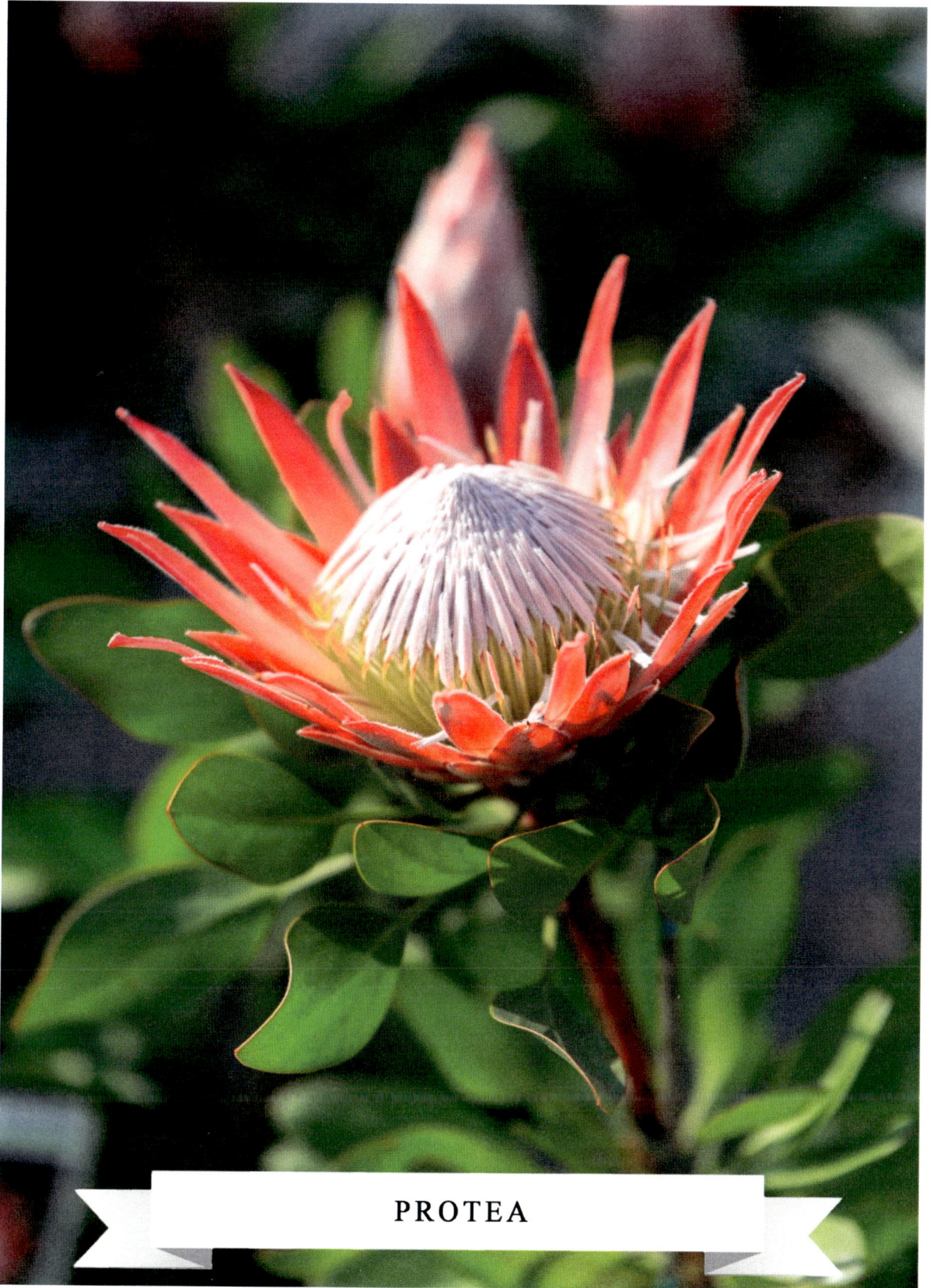

PROTEA

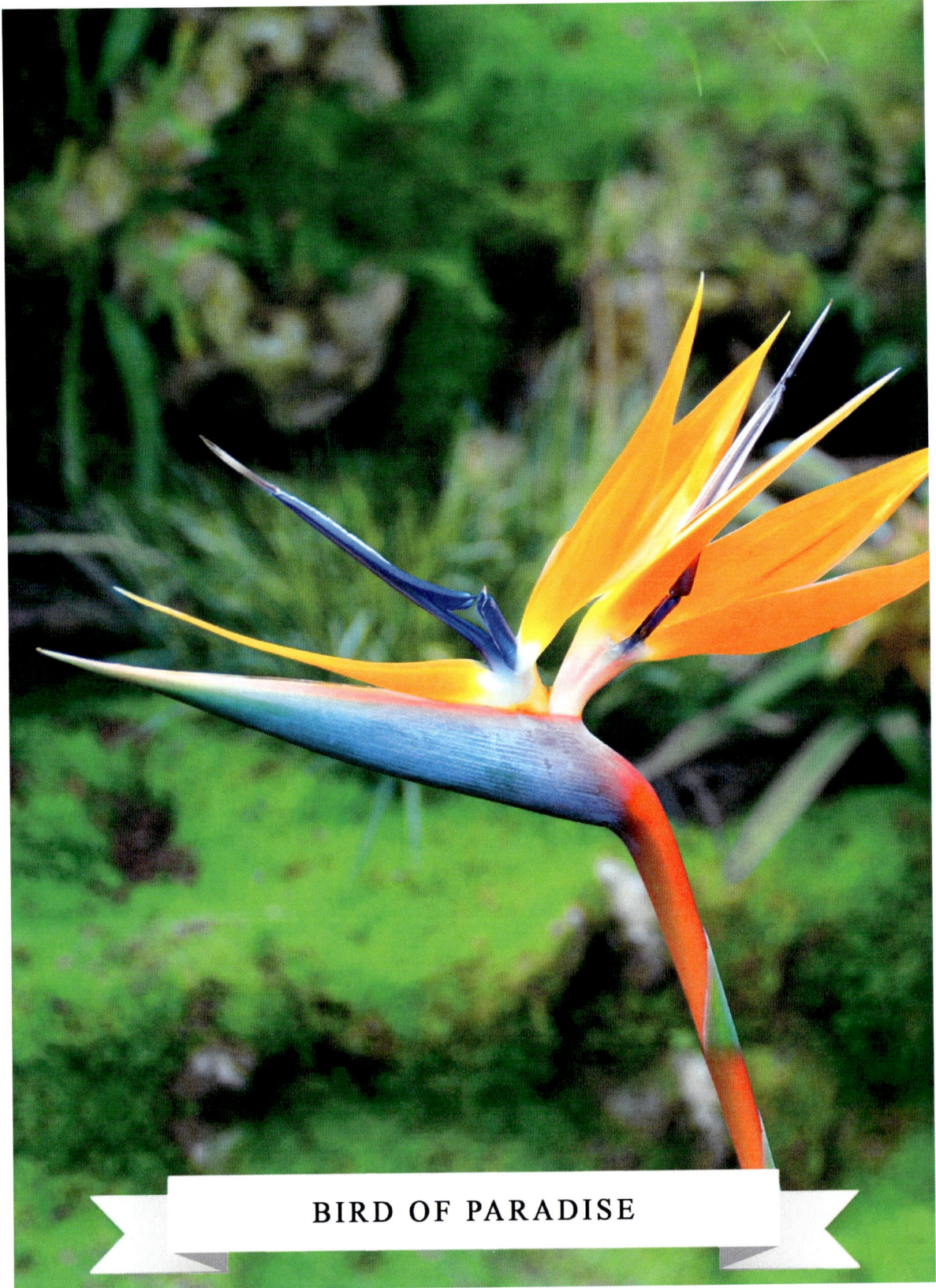

BIRD OF PARADISE

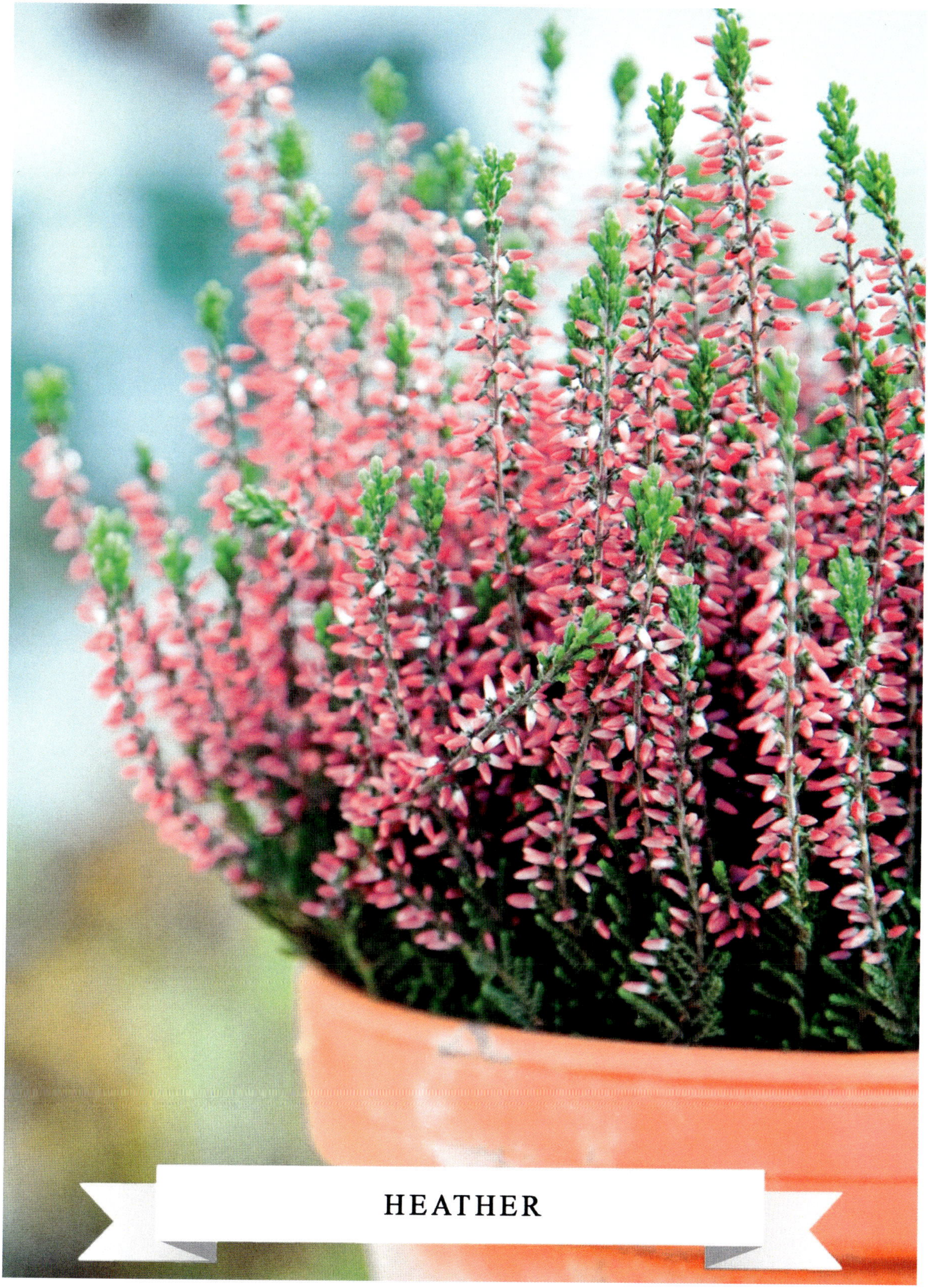

HEATHER

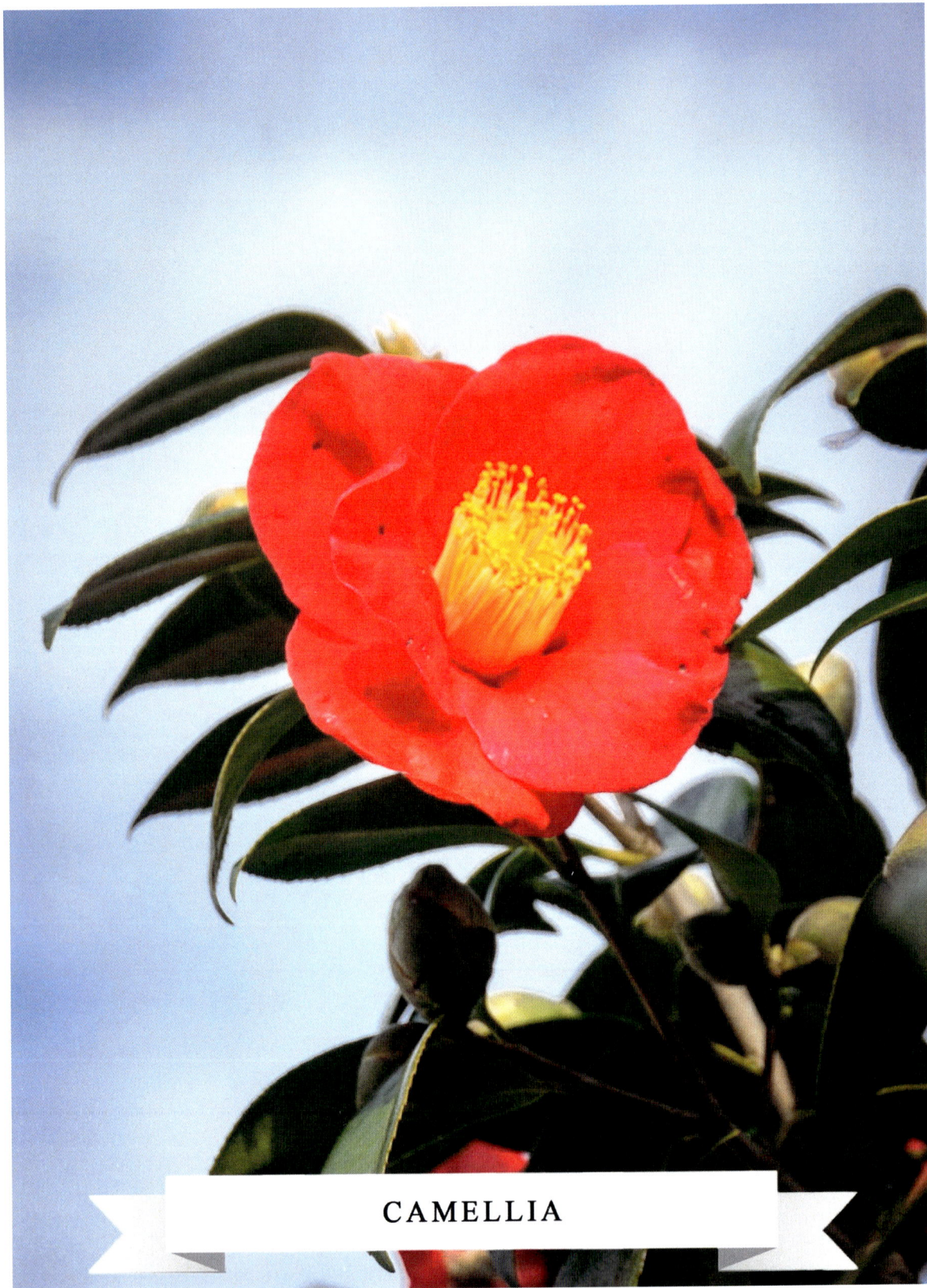

CAMELLIA

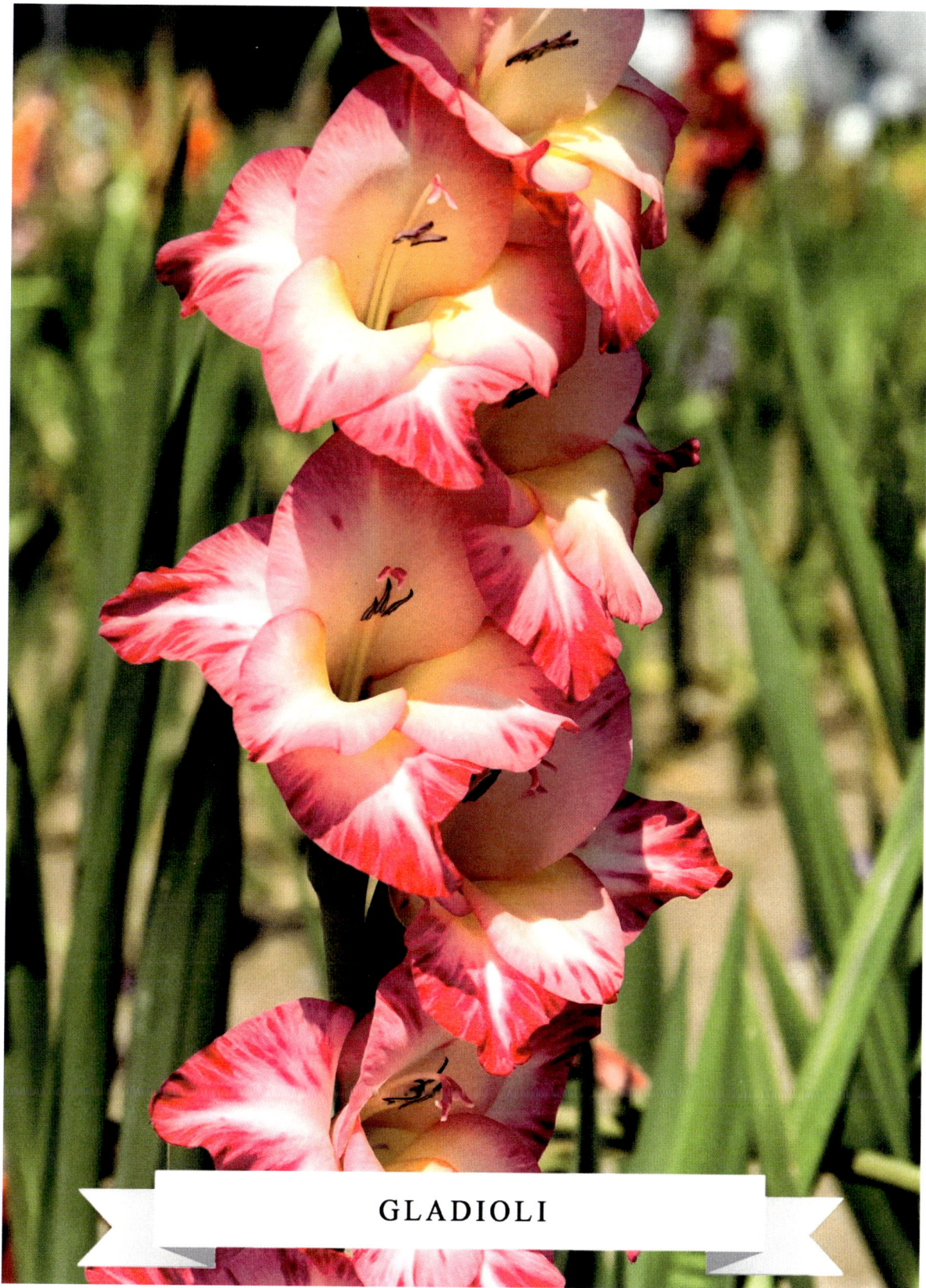

GLADIOLI

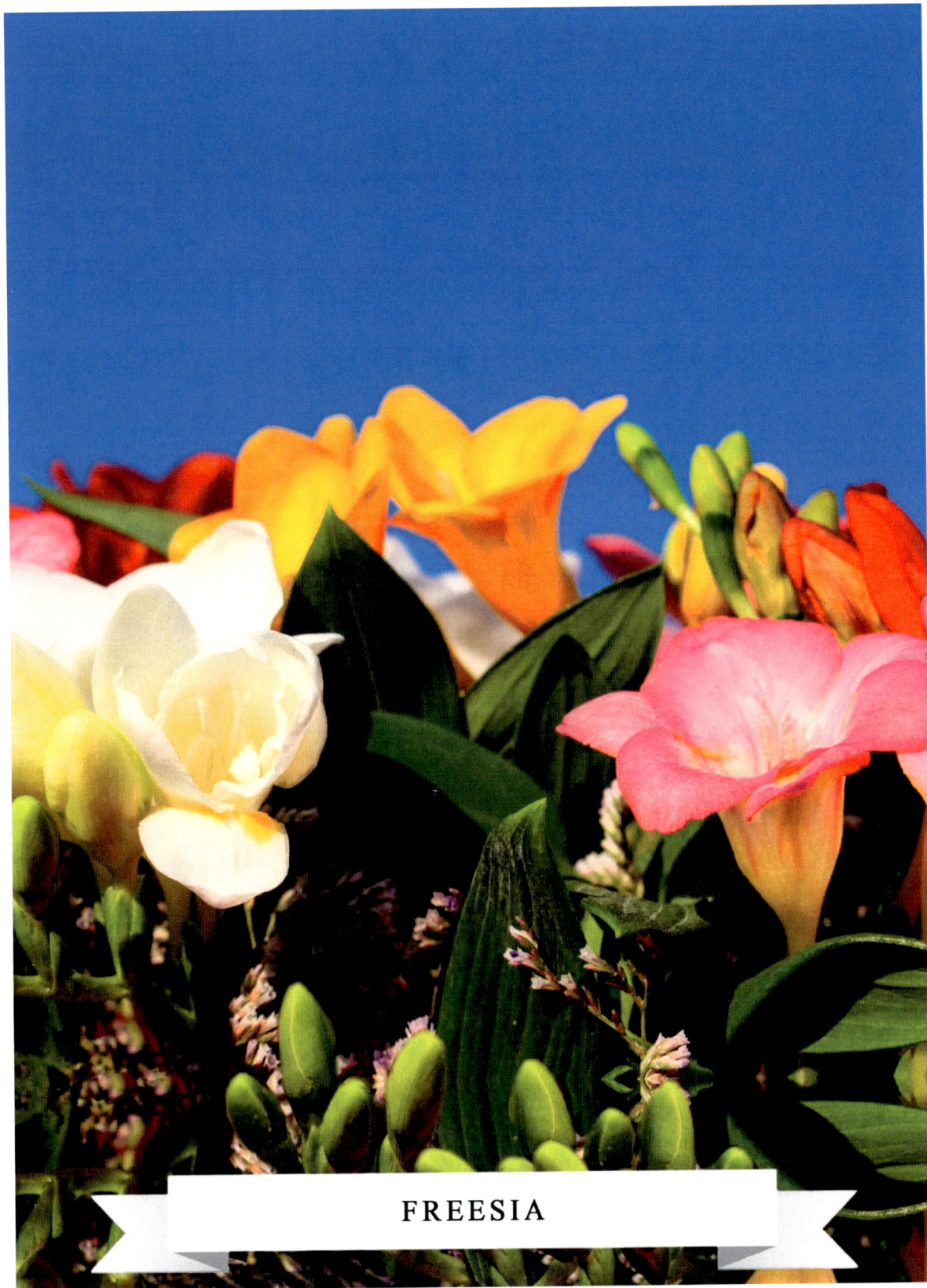

FREESIA

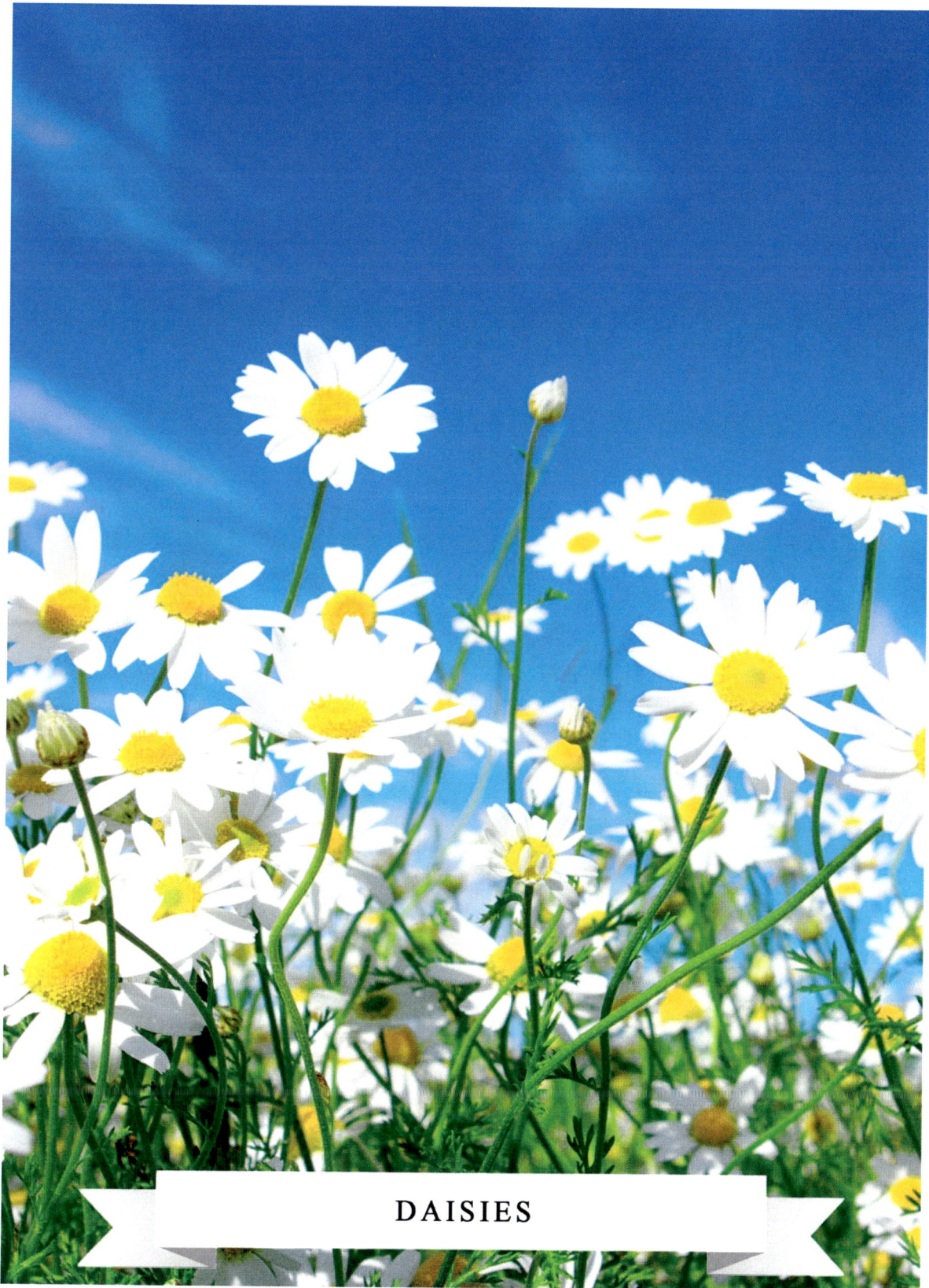

DAISIES

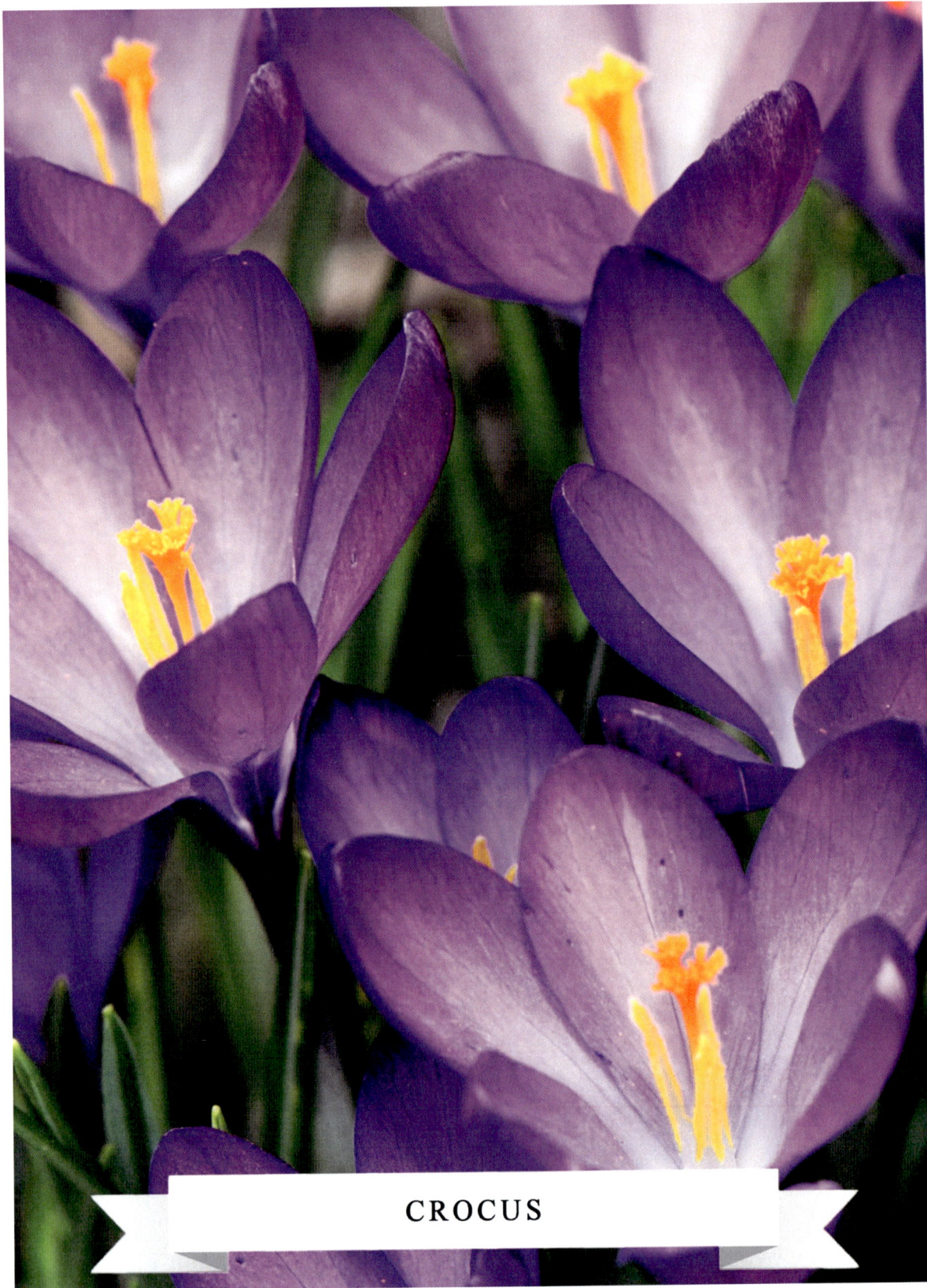

CROCUS

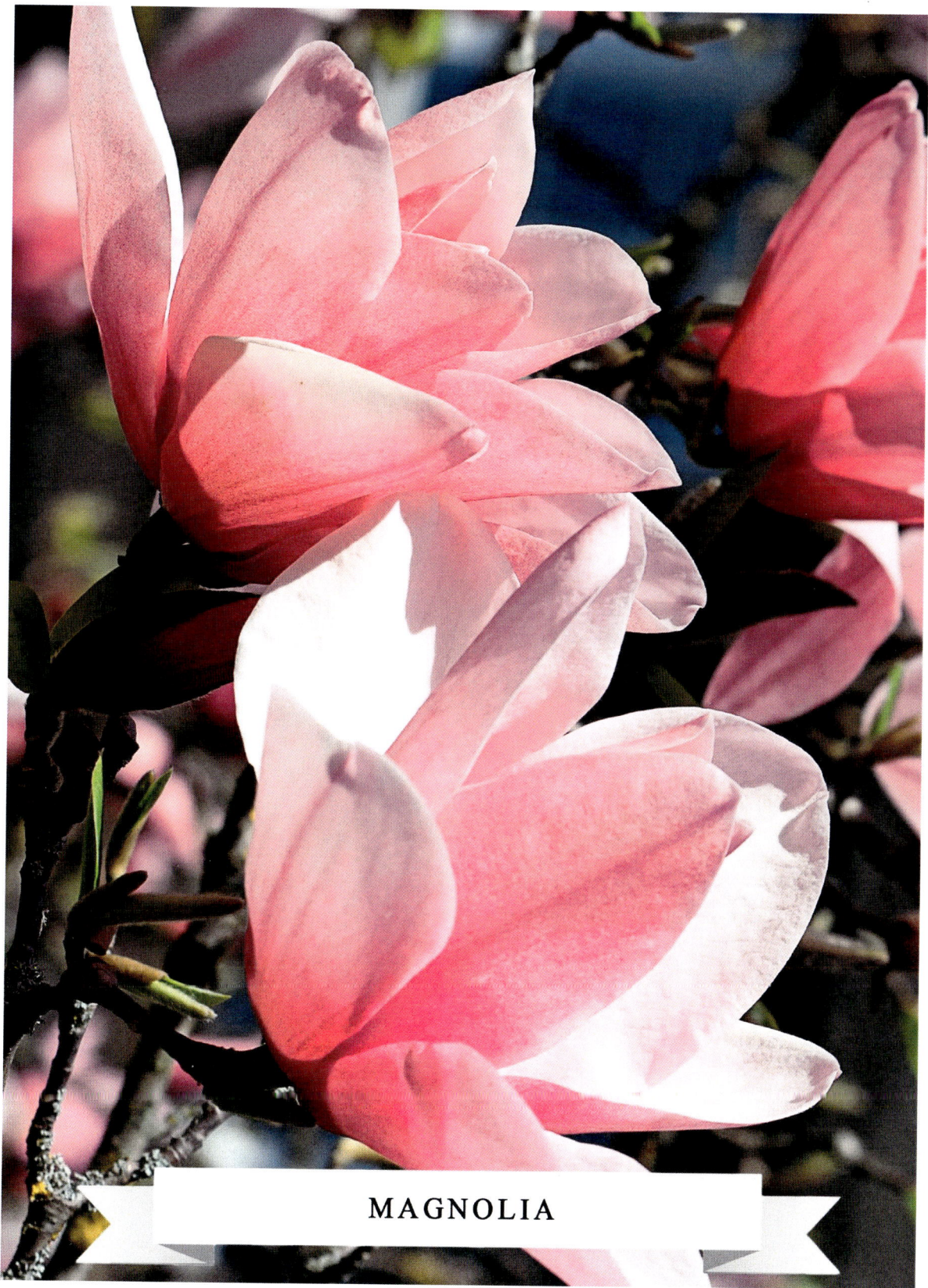

MAGNOLIA

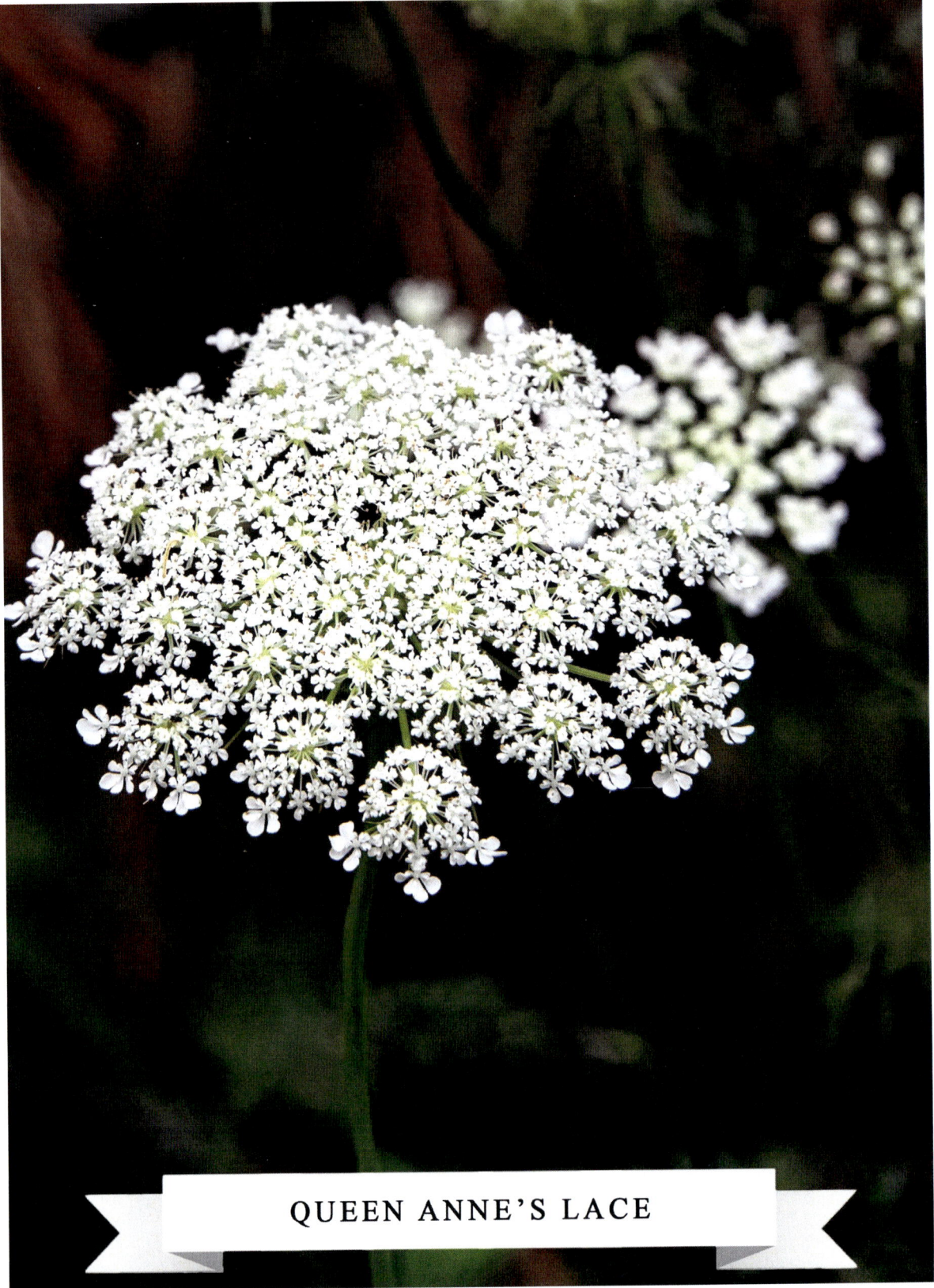

QUEEN ANNE'S LACE

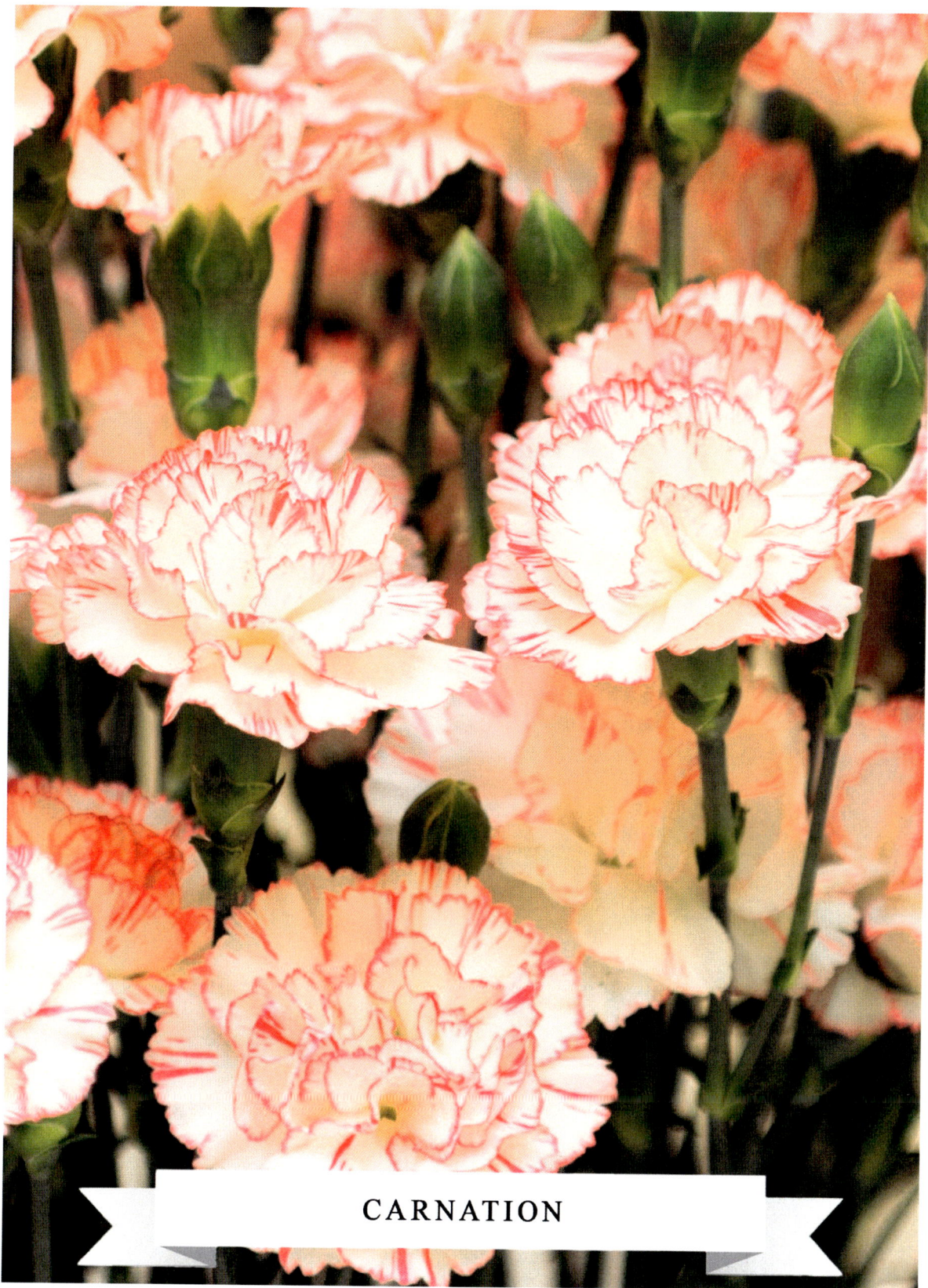

CARNATION

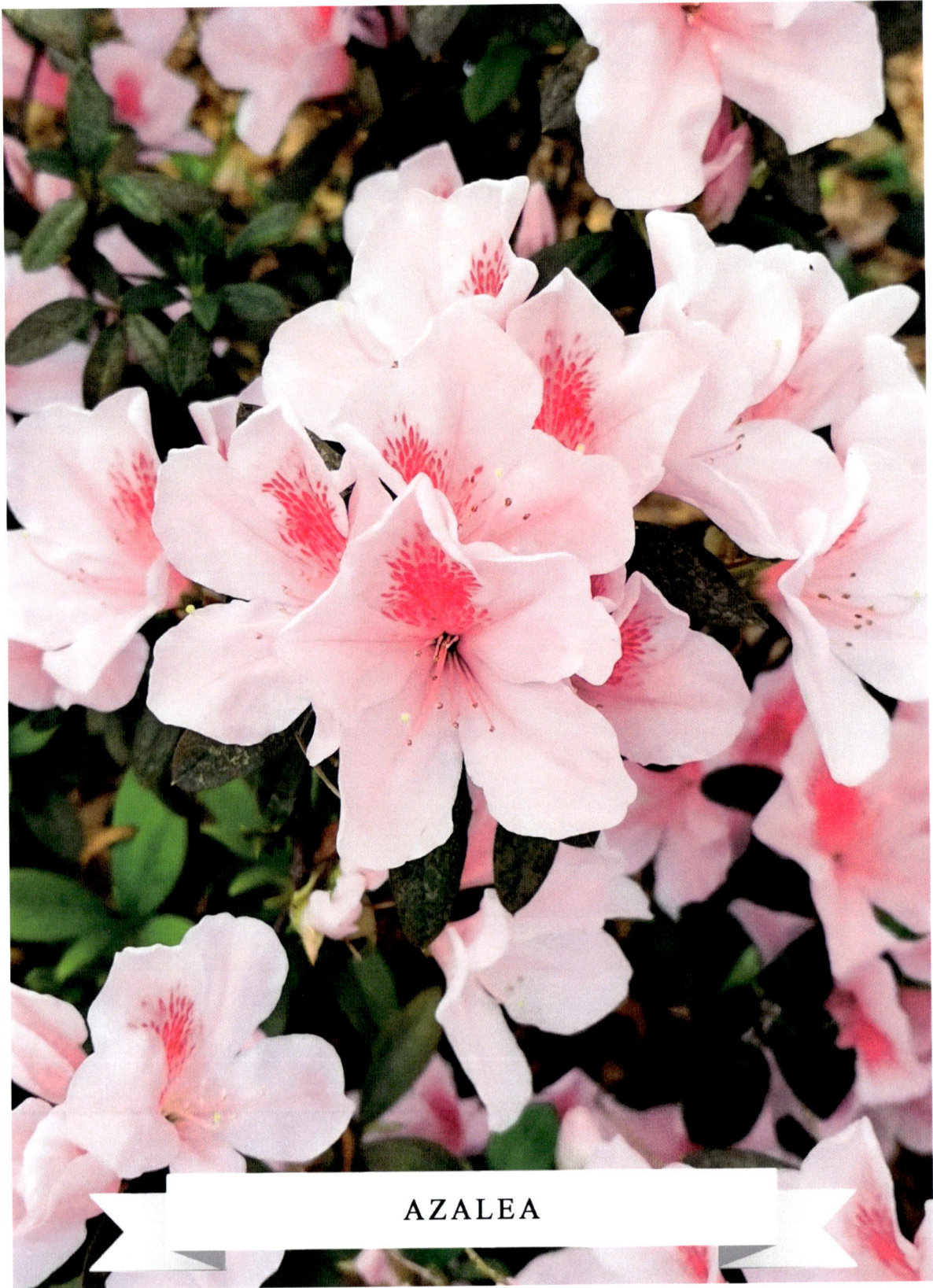

AZALEA

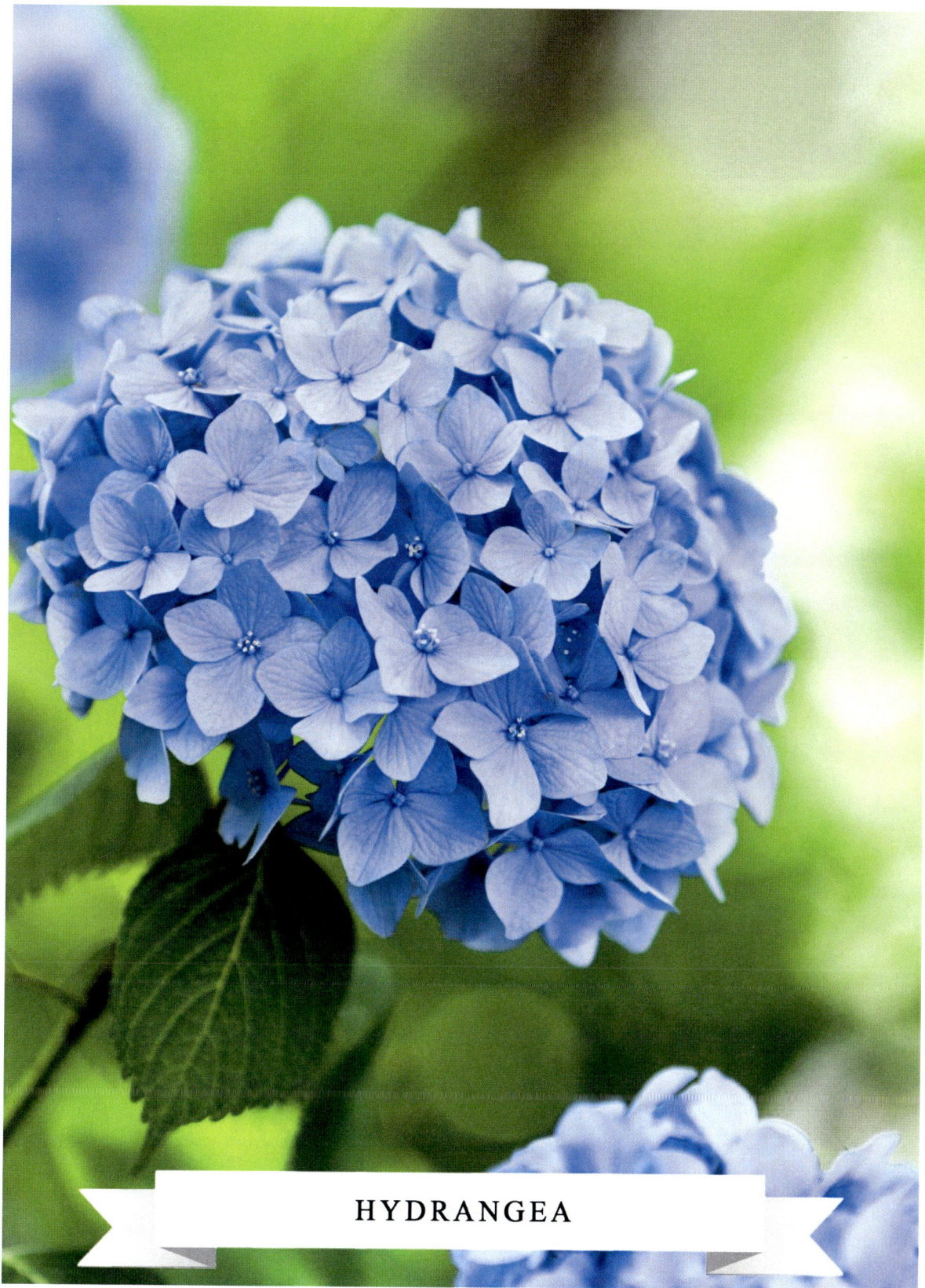

HYDRANGEA

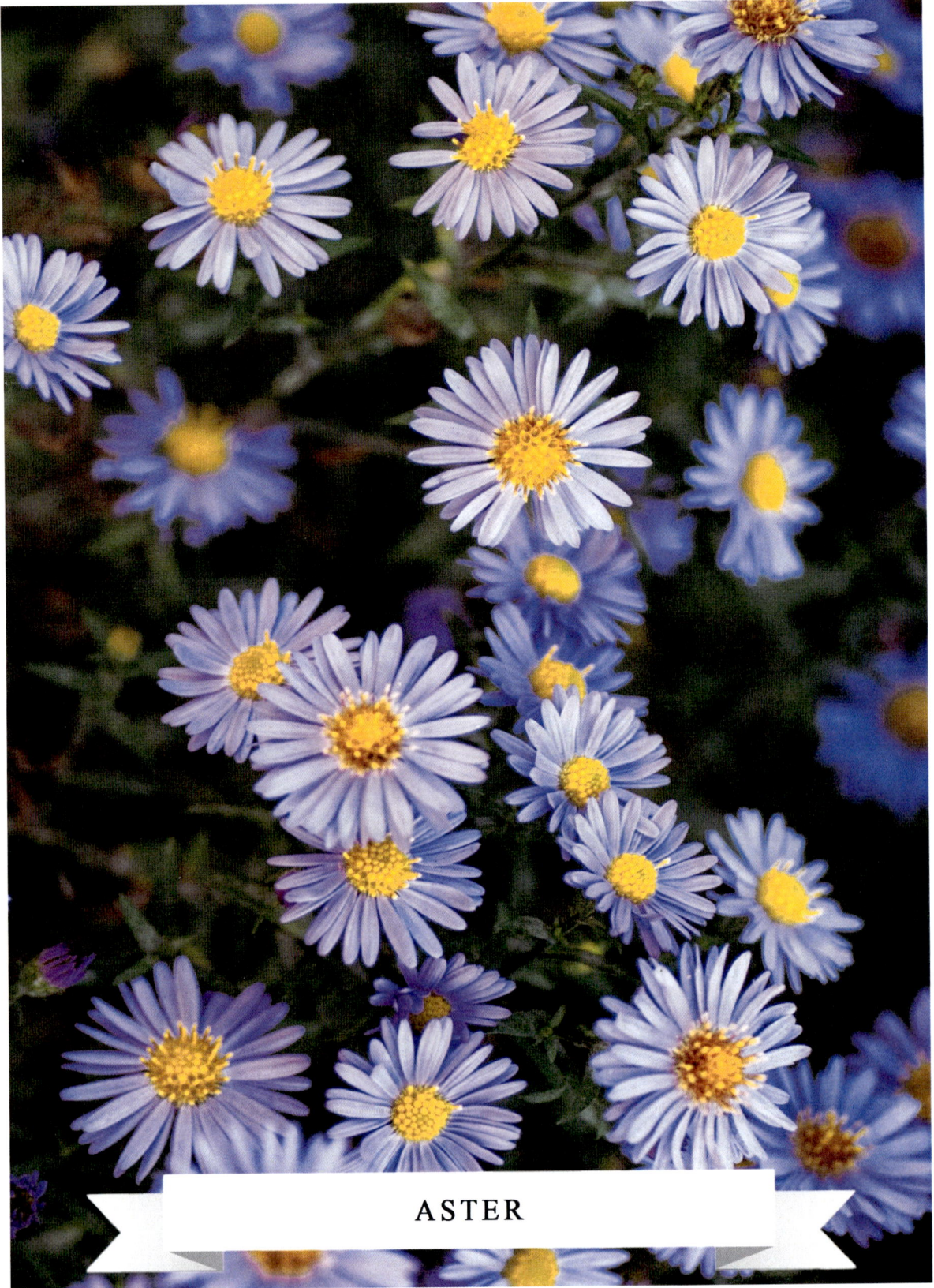

ASTER

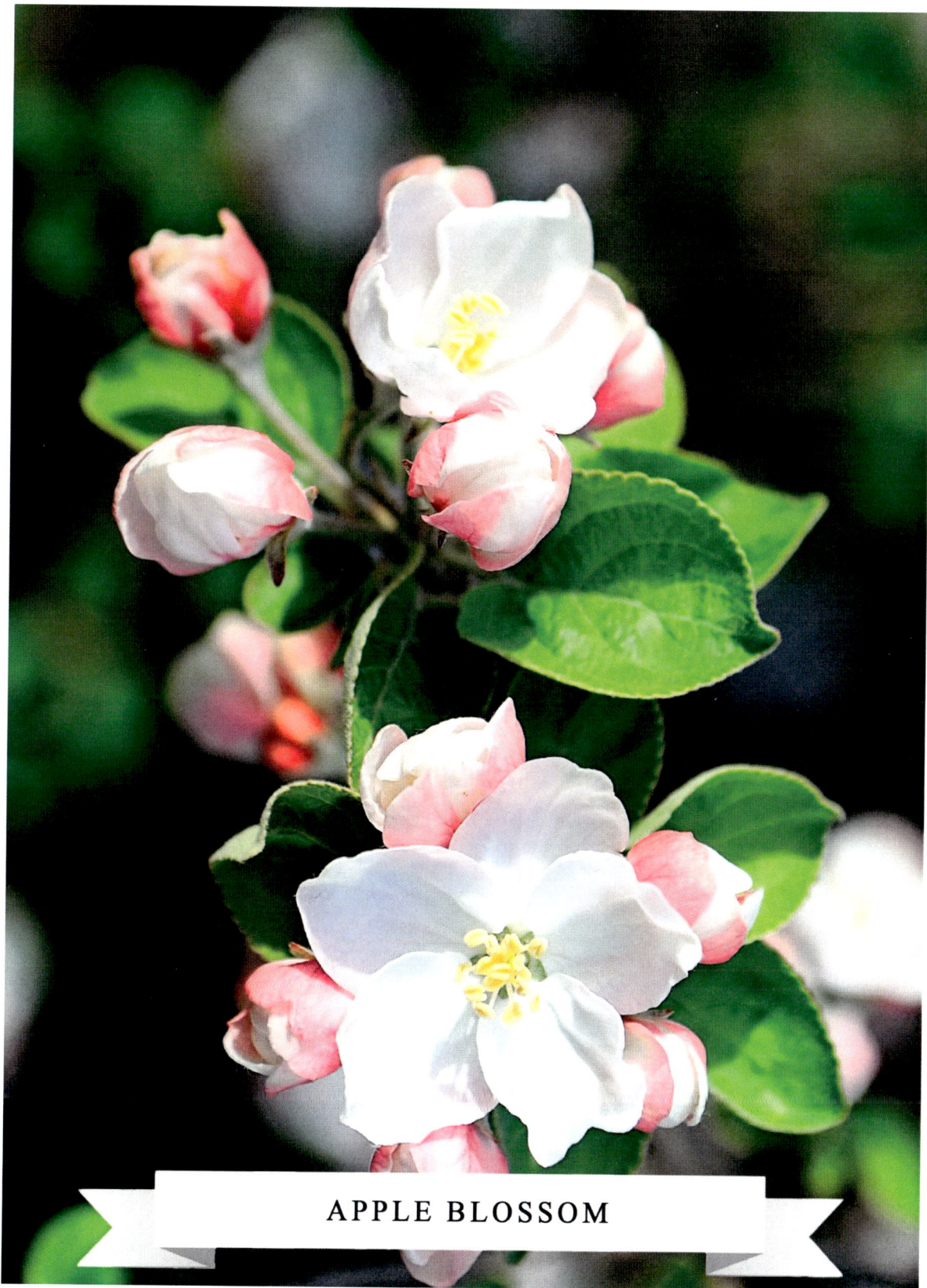

APPLE BLOSSOM

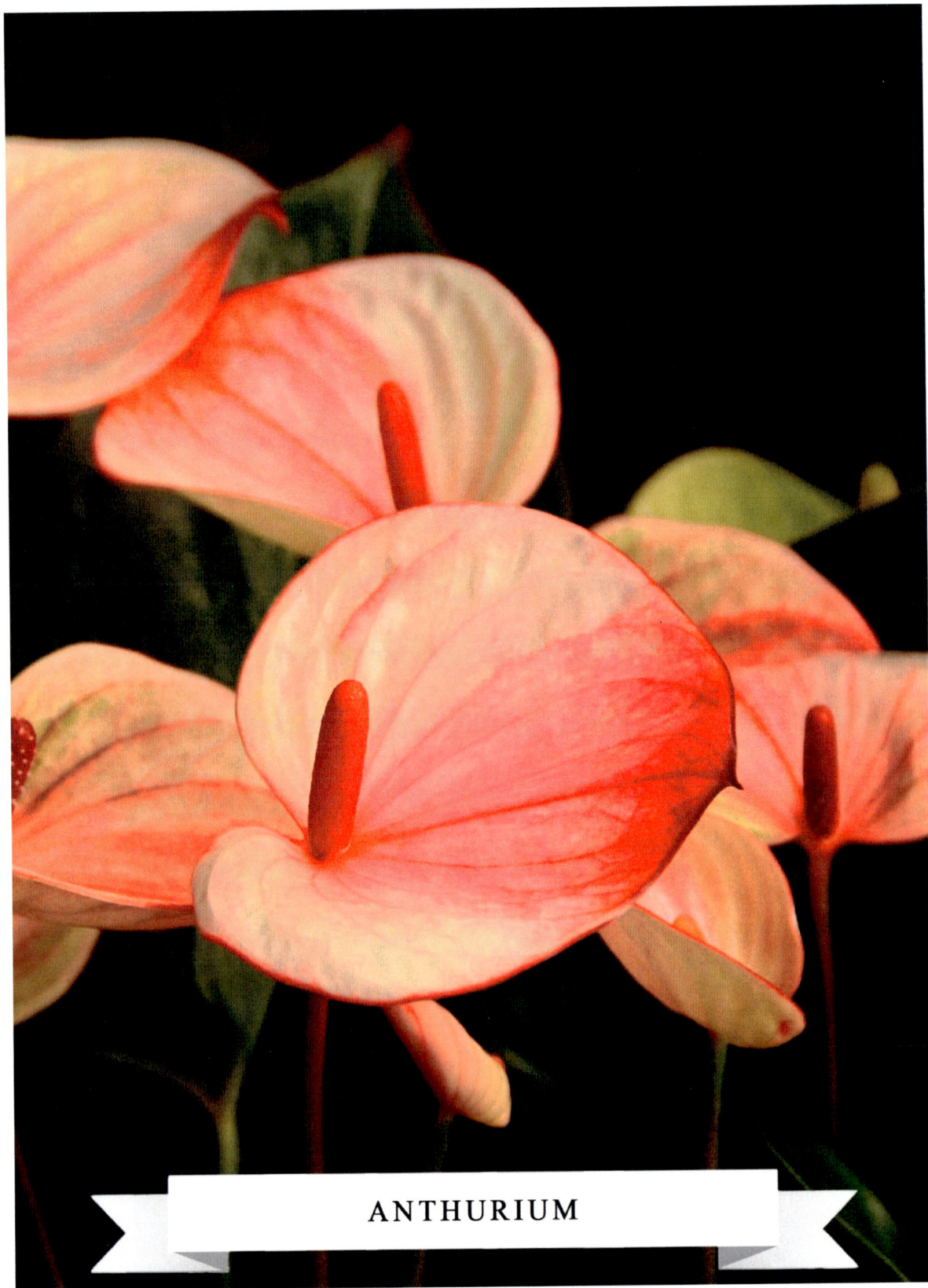

ANTHURIUM

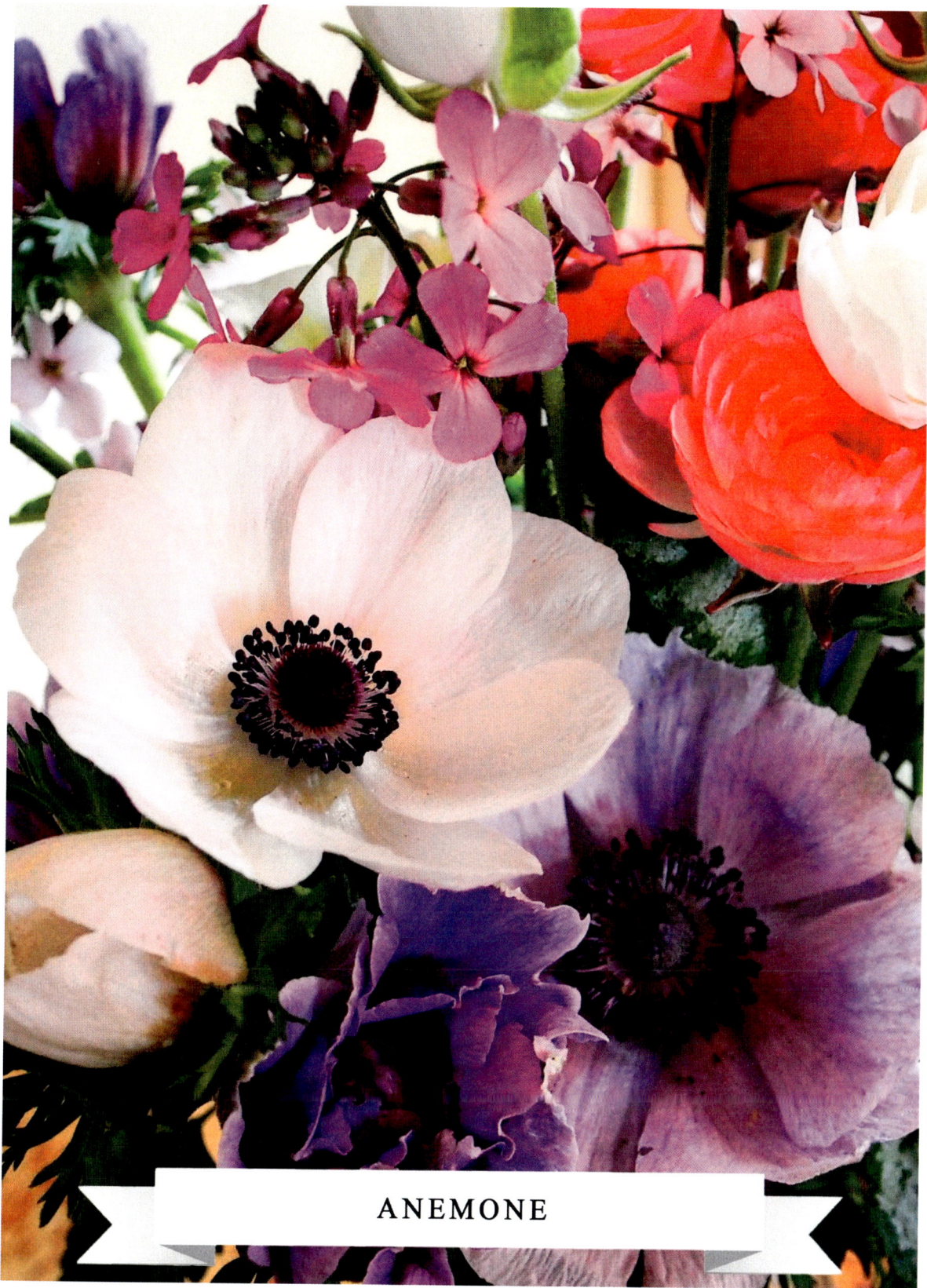

ANEMONE

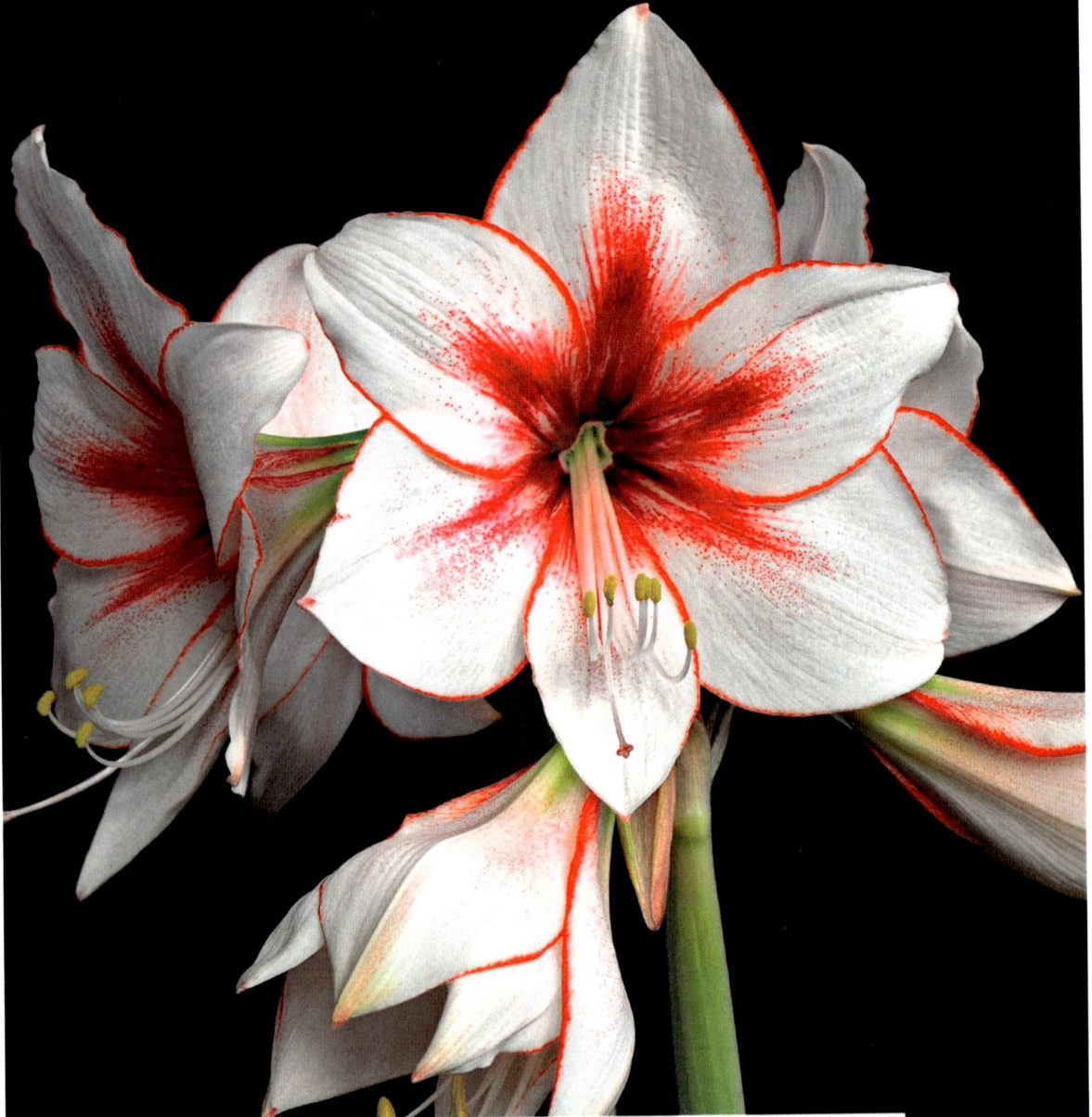

AMARYLLIS

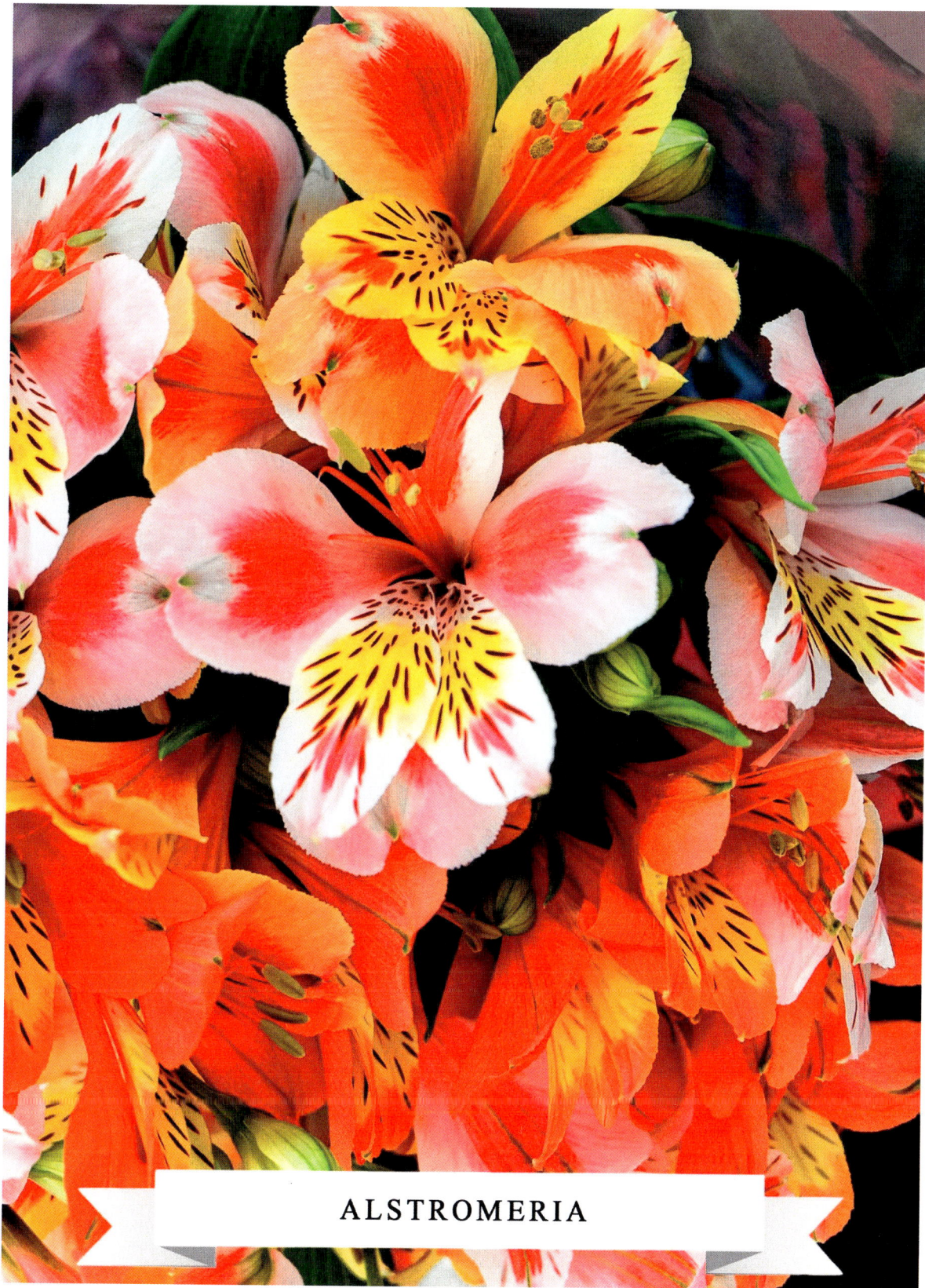

ALSTROMERIA

Thank you

Thanks for your interest in our books.

Please consider purchasing our other books
available now at Amazon.com.

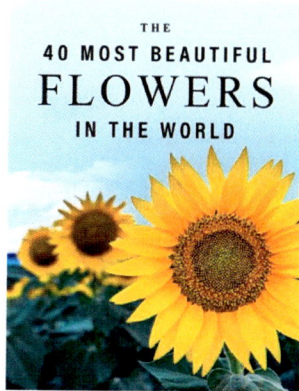

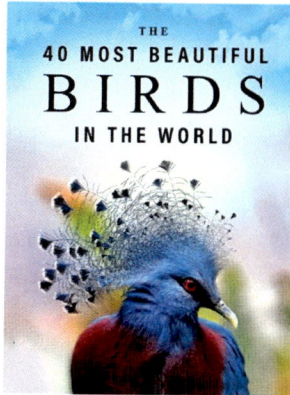

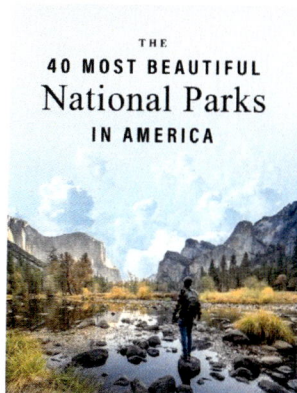

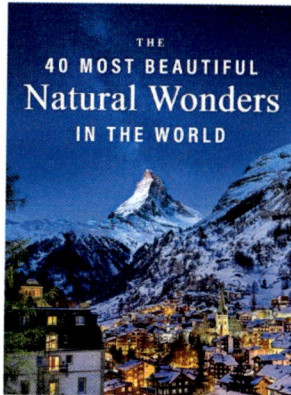

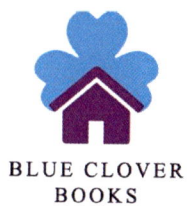

Made in the USA
Monee, IL
02 January 2024

50914186R00026